Developmental Drama

MARY BOOKER

Developmental Drama

Dramatherapy Approaches for
People with Profound or Severe Multiple
Disabilities, Including Sensory Impairment

Jessica Kingsley *Publishers*
London and Philadelphia

First published in 2011
by Jessica Kingsley Publishers
73 Collier Street
London N1 9BE, UK
and
400 Market Street, Suite 400
Philadelphia, PA 19106, USA

www.jkp.com

Library of Congress Cataloging in Publication Data
Booker, Mary.
  Developmental drama : dramatherapy approaches for people with profound or
severe multiple disabilities, including sensory impairment / Mary Booker.
       p. cm.
  Includes bibliographical references and index.
  ISBN 978-1-84905-235-1 (alk. paper)
  1. Drama--Therapeutic use. 2. People with disabilities--Psychology. 3.
People with disabilities--Rehabilitation. 4. Social interaction. I. Title.
  RC489.P7.B55 2011
  617'.0651--dc22
                              2011007674

British Library Cataloguing in Publication Data
A CIP catalogue record for this book is available from the British Library

ISBN 978 1 84905 235 1
eISBN 978 0 85700 478 9

CONTENTS

1

INTRODUCTION AND ACKNOWLEDGEMENTS: WORKING IN THE DARK

Not long after I started working at a special school for children and young people with visual impairment and complex needs, I overheard an exasperated colleague in the staff room say, 'What these children need is to learn how to play!'

She was expressing the frustration she continually faced in trying to help move profoundly disabled, visually impaired children forward in their development. In those early days another experienced member of staff insisted to me that he had seen no evidence of profoundly disabled, visually impaired children having any 'imagination'. For a dramatherapist this was a bit of a red flag to a bull. Children with complex needs have a right to play, just as all children do (Orr 2003) and imagination is fundamental to humanity (Harris 2000). I felt certain that dramatherapy had something to offer these children and young people, but knew it was up to me to find out what before banging my dramatherapy tambourine in the staff room.

That was in 1998. This book is the result of more than ten years' effort to do just that. Along the way, I undertook a master's degree in special education for those with multisensory impairment (MSI, formerly deafblind). I found little written in the field of dramatherapy that directly dealt in any depth with what I needed to know, but I did discover a rich resource of information, wisdom and support within the field of special education. My hope is that this book will begin to fill in the gap in dramatherapy literature concerning this client group.

Before starting at this special school, I already had ten years of dramatherapy experience that included working with adults with learning disabilities and children with a range of special needs. I had occasionally come up against sensory impairment, and was aware that people with a hearing or visual impairment needed special consideration in order to access sessions. I had never worked with a person with MSI. Beyond my early training as a teacher and some general psychology input within my dramatherapy training, I was woefully ignorant of the developmental hurdles confronting my clients with learning disabilities, never mind the additional obstacles facing people with profound multiple learning disabilities and sensory impairment. I worked, as many dramatherapists work, through instinct, intuition, imagination and careful observation. I introduced material I felt might be stimulating, within what I believed to be a containing structure, and then made every effort to be aware of how my clients were responding and what they might be trying to communicate.

That is how I started at the school. The Elemental Play approach outlined in this book was derived from that early work. But more than ever before, I began to feel as if I was working in the dark. It seemed an impossible task to understand my multiply disabled, visually impaired clients' world from their perspective. It was just like wandering around in darkness, reaching out for whatever or whoever might be there and at the same time fearing to reach out, listening for the slightest sound, the smallest clue, about what might be going on. Now and again, some of us would 'find' each other – meet and really connect within the play. This happened often enough to keep me, the young people I worked with and the support staff motivated to continue playing.

But I still hadn't discovered what drama itself really had to offer these clients. While pondering how to move on with this, I came across an interesting and appropriate version of the Native American Hopi creation myth of *Grandmother Spider* (Eliot, Campbell and Eliade 1994) and decided to work with it. We spent a term, all together – me, the young people and the support staff – session after session, literally journeying in the darkness, moving from one level of creation to another. I recognised something worthwhile in this exploration I could share with others and in 2003 I took the myth, and the structures I had developed using it, to a specialist MSI (deafblind) unit to see if these children could also benefit. The responses of both the staff and the children were very encouraging. I began to realise then that I was discovering ways of working that could be valuable to other practitioners. I also began to explore using other classic stories within my work at the school.

Our early group explorations were the first real insight I had into my clients' experience. It was clear to me that the clients would always be my main guides in this journey. Those basic tools of instinct, intuition, imagination and observation have held me in good stead throughout. But they would not have taken me the full distance I have travelled. I needed the experience and expertise of others who also work with these kinds of disabilities, practitioners of all kinds. The contents of this book owe much to others. In particular I want to acknowledge two dramatherapists: Chris Hill and Ian Siddons Heginworth, whose creative and inspirational work with people with learning disabilities was formative in the early years of my work with this client group. I wish to thank Keith Park for his advice and support. He is an inspiring drama practitioner, with deafblind experience, whose ideas on engaging severe and profoundly disabled young people with classical literature through drama have influenced the approaches in this book. I also need to mention Liz Platt, whose personal support and unfailing enthusiasm for Developmental Drama has been invaluable, and Clive Fowler, from whom I learned so much about the needs of young people with profound or severe multiple disabilities and sensory impairment. Special thanks goes to Heather Murdock for the drum warm-up in Chapter 6.

This book is written by a practitioner – for practitioners. It will present the ways I have developed over many years working with children and young people with profound or severe multiple disabilities. My intention is to encourage others to work more confidently and creatively with clients with profound or severe multiple disabilities, including those with sensory impairments. The ideas in this book are not a complete map. They are meant to be a starting point for the reader-practitioner's own journey in this area of work. In addition to dramatherapists, I hope that teachers, who would like to do drama with children with profound or severe multiple disabilities but wonder how to go about it, might also find inspiration within these pages.

2

THE CLIENT GROUP

The client group who inspired the approaches in this book are sometimes referred to as having multiple disabilities and visual impairment (MDVI) or MSI. However, these ways of working can be applicable to the full range of people with profound or severe multiple learning disabilities (PMLD/SLD), including those on the autistic spectrum. Some kind of sensory impairment occurs far more frequently in people defined as having a learning disability than in the general population. The impairment may not necessarily be in the sense organs themselves, but in the parts of the brain that process sensory information. Much of my work has been done with adolescents and young adults (13–21 years), but Developmental Drama can be relevant to any age group, including older people.

Formal assessments of people within these client groups often include the phrase *global developmental delay*. What does this mean and how does it manifest in the individual? And what effect does sensory impairment have on this? Global developmental delay means that the person has been significantly unable to achieve important milestones in all areas of development. People with profound learning disabilities would generally still be at a very early stage of development whatever their age. Within Piaget's (1967) seminal model of development, most would be seen as still operating within the pre-verbal world of the sensory-motor period. Even people with severe learning disabilities who have managed to gain some language skills will experience serious obstacles to continued development. For people with profound or severe disabilities, developmental progress, however slow, is not an orderly process of construction like building with bricks, but there are some important foundations. As with normal infants and children, it relies on the creation of trusting, interactive relationships and the provision of reliable and responsive environments – environments that are engineered to foster development (Ware 2003).

When referring to the development of a human being from conception to fully functioning adult, it is usual to break it into various aspects, for example, physical development, cognitive development, social development, emotional development, language development and so on. Developmental theories tend to centre around one or more of these aspects. This belies the holistic reality of development. All aspects are deeply interconnected and together form a unique, overall developmental process for each individual. Anyone who has worked alongside these clients will know that every person with profound and multiple disabilities is a unique and whole human being, complex and impossible to quantify. They are continuously developing as people, however 'delayed' this might be. Consider Henry who has profound and multiple disabilities including visual impairment. He has little control over his own body, only able to turn his head and slightly move his limbs. When excited his whole body tenses and quivers. Assessment puts him at a developmental level of approximately six months, but this does not mean he is like a baby. Henry is 14 years old and, despite his severely limited physical capacity, he has had many years experience in making and maintaining relationships. He has a distinct personality and also considerable experience in living within the constraints his disabilities have placed him under.

Each individual also has their own unique mix of obstacles to development. These affect social and emotional development, including the development of attachment, as well as cognitive development. There is a bewildering array of possibilities within the range of PMLD/SLD, including:

- A number of medical conditions that may have necessitated the person being hospitalised for frequent and/or long periods, including during the developmentally vital first three years.

- A wide spectrum of physical disabilities that affect physical movement and development from simple coordination problems, through conditions that come under the umbrella of cerebral palsy, to conditions of minimal physical functioning necessitating total physical care, specialist wheelchairs, etc. These also may result in frequent and/or long terms of hospitalisation.

- Sensory disabilities including visual impairment (VI) from mild to total blindness, hearing impairment from mild to total deafness, wide ranges of problems with Sensory Integration similar to those found in people with severe autism, and endless variations on dual sensory impairment (vision and hearing) which has become known as MSI. The effects of MSI go way beyond that of VI or deafness. When both the distance senses are affected, the person can be almost totally deprived of the essential capacity to comprehend what is happening around them and to them.

- Epilepsy, from mild to severe, which can affect cognitive functioning. The frequency and duration of mild epileptic seizures can often be more learning disabling than infrequent but strong seizures.

- Profound cognitive disabilities, meaning that explorative behaviour (including play), comprehension, memory and language development are all seriously affected.

With so many variables and combinations interacting with each other in affecting development, these obstacles can seem overwhelming to those who work with people with profound disabilities. Consider the following children:

Robert is sitting on a cushioned plastic-covered surface in a darkened room. He is facing a lighted tube in which bubbles constantly rise through liquid. His legs are on either side of the tube and his forehead is resting on the tube that gently hums. He pulls away, puts his hands over his ears and makes a vibrating sound with his lips. Then both hands go onto the bubble tube. He vocalises, 'mumumumum.' He taps the right side of his head gently with his fist and then puts his forehead back against the tube surface. His eyes are open, staring at the bubbles. He stays like this, completely still, for 30 seconds or more. Sitting next to him is Anne, an adult he knows well. She speaks near to Robert's ear now and again, but he pays no attention to her. He takes his head away from the tube, closes his eyes and vocalises again, 'yewyewyewyew.' Anne says, 'That's a happy sound!'

In a church hall, less than a mile away, Paul is sitting at a table on which is spread a lovely pile of soapy foam. Sitting across from him is Shirley, an adult he knows well. There are other children playing around him in the hall. He lifts up his two soapy hands to show a girl standing nearby watching him. Then he becomes absorbed in rubbing his hands together. 'Messy hands!' he says. He makes a sound of disgust, but is obviously delighted. He shows the girl again. He claps his hands together and a bit of foam flies onto his nose. He laughs and Shirley laughs. He claps his hands to flick the foam about. Then he looks around to see what is going on in the rest of the room. Returning to his hands, he looks at them. Suddenly he says to Shirley, 'Oh look!' He shows her one of his hands and she looks closely. 'It's your finger!' she says. Then they both leave the table to get cleaned up.

Both of these boys are enjoying an activity with an adult they know well. Beyond that point of similarity, it is the differences that an observer is struck by. Paul is, for all intents and purposes, a normal, lively two and a half year old boy. Robert is six years old. He is a similar size to Paul, but very frail looking by comparison. He was born with a rare genetic condition known as Infantile Refsum's Disease. According to his Statement of Special Educational Needs, this has resulted in him having 'severe physical, sensory and developmental disabilities'. As both Robert's sight and hearing are impaired, he can be referred to as being MSI.

Paul is seen actively exploring the physical environment and interacting with other people. He observes the material he is exploring and the effect his activity has on it. He experiments and, when he finds something he likes doing, repeats and expands on it. He is aware of the people around him and notices the effects his activity has on them. He communicates with sounds, words, gestures and whole body activity. He can share his feelings and experience with others. He is able to gain the attention of the adult he is with when he wants to. He also moves freely from one activity to another.

Cognitively, physically and socially, Paul demonstrates an appropriate developmental level for his age. He is no longer the relatively helpless baby he was at birth. He has matured physically and he has changed in the way he thinks and behaves through a process of active and largely self-motivated learning. He is progressively building on the information he is taking in through his senses from the things and people in his environment, creating and developing working concepts about them. He is energetically interacting with objects and people, creating a sense of an autonomous self in relationship with his world. And he is developing language that will further enhance his concept building, his sense of self and his relationships with others.

Robert is over twice Paul's age. He has no conventional language, only vocalisations. Many of these appear to be self-stimulation rather than overt communications. One has to know him very well to interpret these sounds as having any meaning at all. When he is concentrating on using the little sight he has, he does not appear to attend to sounds. When he is attending to sounds or tactile experiences, he generally closes his eyes. He is mostly wrapped up in the world of his own body, with the sounds and sensations he can create within that sphere. There is little interaction with the objects and people in his environment. They have to come to him rather than him moving out actively to explore. Even then he may retreat from interaction. Because he is not getting the sensory feedback that we take for granted, he has little motivation to expand on his activity, beyond his bodily self-stimulation. He does not have much awareness of the social 'others' around him, and therefore will have little sense of himself as a 'self' in relationship with others. He has little power to alter his own circumstances except by becoming distressed. Just how he does experience the world is impossible for others to truly comprehend, and he cannot communicate his experience. It seems likely that the world outside his own body-sphere either does not exist for him, or feels highly unpredictable and chaotic. He is unable to construct meanings and predictions in the way that normal children do through the integration of their sensory experiences, their interactions and their development of language. This will maintain his passive, withdrawn attitude – or lead to fear and distressed behaviour. Without intervention, he cannot actively learn and develop. His psychological and social development has been hugely curtailed through his disabilities. Robert is not a 'typical' person with profound and multiple disabilities. These clients cannot be typified. But Robert gives us a sense of the difficulties that can be encountered when trying to work with this client group.

Research has shown that children aged two are already able to engage in complex imaginative joint play (Harris 2000), but the interactive cues they require to do this are largely visual, supported by language. This puts children with visual impairment or multi-sensory impairment at a huge disadvantage. When this is combined with other disabilities, the barrier to play is enormous. It is easy to imagine Paul enjoying drama, engaging fully with story and enactment. The challenge here is to explore how to enable a person like Robert to first engage with, and then develop through, drama. In dramatherapy with this client group, therapeutic aims tend to focus on social and emotional development, including communication development. They are about people with PMLD/SLD becoming more aware of themselves and others, especially in terms of how they and others are feeling and how this is expressed and understood. But this is not to separate these aspects from physical and cognitive development. Drama is an invaluable tool for helping with the development of things like cause and effect, exploration of objects and sequencing. The beauty of Developmental Drama, as an OFSTED inspector commented after observing one of our *Grandmother Spider* sessions, is that all aspects of development are worked with together, naturally, within the dramatic experience.

3

THE AIMS OF DEVELOPMENTAL DRAMA

Developmental Drama assumes a holistic stance. As such, it works with the whole person – on many levels and areas at once – acknowledging the interconnectedness inherent in human development. It aims to promote the mental health and development of the person by enabling them to:

- express themselves in response to what is happening within and around them in the session, and know that their expression has been received, understood and valued – in other words, communicate with others

- experience their input as having an effect on the events and people within the session

- gain a sense of what is happening in order to form meanings, develop anticipation and participate to their fullest within the session

- feed their imagination with accessible sensory experiences and images, within meaningful contexts

- encounter and deal with new situations and challenges within the session, discovering new resources within themselves

- develop their emerging emotional intelligence.

Developmental Drama is a social experience. It is about being, learning and developing together in a social and dramatic context rather than about achieving tasks or 'doing' drama. It is a process-orientated way of working. Process is understood as everything that is going on inside each person, between people and within the group as a whole while engaged in an activity. It is the change that happens within individuals and within the group over time – whether that time is a few seconds, an hour, a year or a lifetime. It can be useful to think of it as the dance – in contrast to the steps. Development and therapy are processes. In Developmental Drama it is not the story or the props or the action that is the focus of the therapy. Rather it is the process that happens within and around these activities. Development happens as a result of the processes of the session rather than the content. The process both contains and penetrates the activities within the session. The content is essential however – it is the vehicle for the process.

PLAY

Developmental Drama aims to be fun, absorbing, exciting, intrinsically meaningful and satisfying for everyone involved. This sounds like play. Play lies at the heart of Developmental Drama, just as it is at the heart of human development, creativity and drama. Events that happen in a session can be designed to be both safe and emotionally challenging at the same time. Here the participants are '*free... from normal consequences*' as are children at play (Garvey 1990, p.6). They can cross a stormy sea to face and fight a monster! So, how can people with PMLD/SLD learn to play? Finding answers to this lies first in understanding how play normally develops, and then in creating ways to support this same development for people with PMLD/SLD through the dramatic medium.

Humans are social beings and we learn about ourselves and our environment in the context of our relationships with others. To be assisted by others is a natural part of normal development. To achieve the aims of Developmental Drama we need to enable the client to engage in play at their own developmental level, while also supporting them to play at a slightly higher level. Where the dramatherapist needs to be working with the client is in what Vygotsky (1978) termed *the zone of proximal development* – the space encompassing what someone can already do independently and what they could manage to do either alongside others or with the direct assistance of others. If the process is pitched outside either end of this spectrum, opportunities for learning and development will be reduced.

When a process is designed within the zone of proximal development, with the intention of supporting a person to become progressively more autonomous and to develop skills, confidence and expertise, it is called *scaffolding*. Scaffolding, as a way of helping people learn and develop competence in new skills, is relatively well-known within education (Wood 1998), but less understood and used within dramatherapy. The very image of scaffolding is one of support during a building process that can be removed once the internal structure is strong enough to stand on its own. Supportive scaffolding is recommended to teaching and support staff as a way for them to help children with attachment difficulties find the confidence to begin to explore news ways of behaving and relating with others (Bombèr 2007). The concept of scaffolding is central to effective dramatherapy with people who have profound or severe learning difficulties complicated by physical and sensory impairment.

THE ROLE OF PRIMARY CAREGIVERS IN PLAY DEVELOPMENT

From the initial level of simple responsiveness, responding to stimuli from within and without, a baby begins to use whatever abilities he or she has to make sense of experiences. The social others in the baby's life, generally the main caregivers, initiate a process of gentle and playful interaction on the basis of the baby's responsiveness. As interaction becomes established and elaborated on, social, emotional and communication development proceeds (Stern 2002). The caregivers are not consciously working at development; they are simply enjoying being with the baby. This is basic play – natural and powerful. It happens within a safe, supportive, affectionate relationship. Primary caregivers who actively play with their baby or toddler help them engage in developmentally higher levels of play. They create simple games from the infant's natural behaviours and then develop these games into increasingly diverse and complex games. By being an enthusiastic play partner, they are also modelling the value and pure enjoyment of play.

Because of the obstacles that have been put in the way of their development, people with PMLD, whatever their age, still need the kind of interaction found in this early one-to-one relationship to further their development (Nind and Hewett 2005). The Elemental Play approach outlined later in this book is based on the processes found within mother/infant interaction, but it can, and should, become a natural part of all dramatherapy with clients with PMLD.

THE ROLE OF OTHER CHILDREN IN PLAY DEVELOPMENT

As well as having similar benefits to playing with mother, siblings and other older children also support play development by involving the younger child in their own play. The young child may not 'understand' all that is happening, but they sense the atmosphere of play and they naturally feel the desire to be a part of whatever is going on. Older children will be doing a variety of things that pull the younger ones into the actions of dramatic play (Garvey 1990). They may:

- assign them a character role (e.g. passenger on a train), then speak to them from their own play role (train conductor) and address them as if they were the assigned role ('*Show me your ticket, please*')

- make explicit play transformations (e.g. line up chairs and then say, '*This is a train!*')

- describe on-going actions (e.g. '*The train is coming into a station. It's slowing down. We're here now. You can get off the train*')

- comment on characters' feelings and what they will do next (e.g. '*You're tired from your long train ride. Let's go to a café!*').

In order for people with PMLD to learn to play, those who work with them need to both play with them as a mother plays with her infant *and* play with them as another, slightly older child might play with them. This second kind of play becomes especially important when working with SLD clients. The aims stated at the start of this chapter also require this play to be carefully designed to take account of the disabilities the clients have, while maximising their abilities. One of those aims is the development of emotional intelligence. Alongside understanding play development, we need to understand what emotional intelligence is, and how it can be developed.

4

THE DEVELOPMENT OF EMOTIONAL INTELLIGENCE

Psychological theory in the United States during the 1980s and 1990s expanded the view of intelligence beyond IQ criteria by including the affective aspect of the mind, referred to as emotional intelligence (EQ). It is a way of thinking that is evaluative in nature (Greenspan 2001). It enables us to really respond appropriately to our environment and develop our interaction with it.

The emotionally intelligent person is able to *perceive* emotions in themselves and others, *understand* those emotions, *regulate* them and *use* them positively and creatively to enhance their lives (Mayer and Salovey 1997). When working with people with PMLD/SLD, especially combined with sensory impairment, enabling our clients to achieve all this seems insurmountable. Yet a large part of human communication is emotional communication, and communication development for people with PMLD focuses on affective responses (O'Kane and Goldbart 1998). It is where we must start.

Emotional intelligence develops both over time (maturation) and through experience (learning). The specific development of emotional intelligence has come to be known as 'emotional literacy'. Goleman (1996 citing Mayer and Salovey 1990) describes five 'domains' within EQ:

- Knowing one's emotions – self-awareness.

- Managing emotions.

- Motivating oneself.

- Empathy.

- Handling relationships.

These domains interact with and support each other, and can all be worked on within Developmental Drama. Let's start by looking at motivation and empathy.

MOTIVATION AND ATTENTION

Motivation is a key ingredient in emotional intelligence – feeling positive and wanting to participate and move forward in life. Goleman (1996) makes two points about motivation that are relevant to Developmental Drama. One concerns the motivating value of cultivating a positive attitude towards oneself as an aspect of EQ. The other is the concept of 'flow', which also affects motivation. Goleman describes flow as 'the ultimate in harnessing the emotions in the service of performance and learning' (1996, p.90). It is a state characterised by both *attention* (focused awareness) and *absorption* (self-forgetfulness) that enables high levels of performance and satisfaction. It results from a combination of mastery (confidence in one's skills and abilities) and a sense of challenge that is stretching. This relates to Buck's (1986) discussion of 'emotional aliments' and 'accessibility' when applying Piaget's theory of cognitive development to emotional development. A task must create a sufficient level of possibility for assimilation but not too much, thus providing a challenge and motivation to learn. Goleman maintains that if you are 'moved' by something – really engaged – you will learn without effort. Therefore, our PMLD/SLD clients in dramatherapy need to:

- experience themselves as valued and celebrated members of the group

- develop confidence in their ability to participate

- heighten their attention to a point of absorption in the activity

- feel challenged to a level that motivates them to stay with the process.

In Chapter 6 we will look at structures that can enable these things.

EMPATHY

Empathy can be said to develop in four stages (Hoffman 1987 cited in Schaffer 1996). The first three of these are relevant to Developmental Drama. The initial stage is a kind of spontaneous *mirroring*, or motor mimicry, seen in infants within the first year. In their undifferentiated state, babies will respond to the distress of another by crying themselves. They will smile or laugh when their mother smiles or laughs to them. This early physical mirroring of another's feelings is essential as it takes empathy into the realm of shared emotional experience, rather than more distanced 'sympathetic' thoughts. Real empathy is not just awareness of another having feelings or a reaction to another's emotions. It involves the capacity for an 'as if' experience of another's emotional state that promotes a sense of understanding and connection with them (Goleman 1996). To get to this point is a long journey for our PMLD/SLD clients, but our task is to help them move towards it.

As the infant develops, the range and subtlety of the emotions they can mirror expands. A developing 'sense of self' within the second year of life brings about the next stage of *egocentric empathy*. It is during this time that children begin to intentionally comfort other people (Harris 1989). Children become aware that it is the 'other', and not themselves, expressing the emotion, but still assume the reason for the emotion is the same as it would be for them. A toddler, for instance, may generously offer their teddy to a baby who is crying because it is hungry. Gradually, the child becomes aware that the teddy is not what the crying baby needs – that *others have their own reasons for expressing emotion*. This kind of understanding constitutes the third stage and develops in the third year of life, enabling the child to offer more appropriate help. The spontaneous emotional response of a two or three-year-old child to another's emotional expression may not be as sophisticated and generalised as an adult's, but it can have all the hallmarks of real empathy.

In terms of our clients, the problem with Hoffman's model of empathy development is that it assumes the distance senses are intact, that sensory information is able to be processed and there has been no disruption to the development of secure attachment. It is the distance senses of vision and hearing that are used to detect the emotional state of another. The facial expressions of others can be unavailable to our clients, and the sounds others make may be difficult for them to make sense of.

Goleman also claims that calm and receptivity in a person are essential to empathy. A person needs to feel secure enough in themselves, before they can take on board, and respond to, the emotional state of others. Therefore, when providing an environment in Developmental Drama where the seeds of empathy might grow, care needs to be taken to:

- enable the emotional state of others to be as accessible as possible to the client's available senses

- develop sufficient safety and calm within the situation for the client to be receptive to the emotions of another.

The environment influences the development of empathetic concern, and young children explore 'hurting' as well as comforting (Harris 1989). Any attempt to intentionally promote empathy development will need to provide the kind of environment necessary to normal empathy development that:

- satisfies the child's own emotional needs, but discourages excessive self-concern

- encourages the child to identify, experience and express a broad range of emotions and

- provides numerous opportunities to observe other people's emotional responsiveness (Barnet 1987 cited in Schaffer 1996, p.179).

Without empathy – being able to emotionally imagine ourselves in another's shoes – we could not emotionally engage in the 'dramatic paradox' at the heart of dramatic play and, according to Robert Landy (1993), also at the heart of dramatherapy. The dramatic paradox is that a person can, at the same time as being themselves, be in the state of 'as if' they were another. It is a simultaneous experience of two different identities that blend together. Children engaged in dramatic play know it is pretend, but that doesn't make it any the less intense and real for them.

There are connections between empathy, play and pretence – and, therefore, drama (Garvey 1990; Sherratt and Peter 2002). Research shows how infants' early affective interaction with others promotes the development of both symbolic play and an understanding of the mental/emotional states of others (Hobson *et al*. 1997). It is the activation of the imagination that produces an empathetic response. Harris (1989, p.52) heralds the imagination as 'a key that unlocks the minds of other people and allows the child temporarily to enter into their plans, hopes and fears'. If Developmental Drama provides the kind of environment described above, it can begin to stimulate and feed the imagination, broadening the PMLD/SLD client's experience beyond the normal possibilities of their everyday reality, both in terms of emotional expression and emotional scenarios.

Our clients with profound or severe learning disabilities are likely to be somewhere in the first or second stages of empathy development. Within a scaffolded approach, some can also work towards the third stage. There are important emotional skills that are contingent to and provide on-going support for the growth of empathy. This takes us into the three other domains of emotional intelligence mentioned at the beginning of this chapter, and requires us to look at general emotional development within the first two years of life. It must always be remembered that our clients are usually much older than this and, for instance, the hormones of adolescence can mean that some aspects of their development are at odds with other aspects.

KNOWING ONE'S EMOTIONS: EXPERIENCING AND IDENTIFYING

Most studies done to identify and measure emotions as they first appear in infants rely entirely on the infant's intact vision – being able to *see* the face of another. However, this research can inform us by providing some answers to the questions:

- What are emotions?

- How do they develop?

- How do we learn to know them?

Emotions are notoriously subjective and yet are almost universally understood (Harris 1989). Bullock and Russell (1986, p.203) claim that emotions are not technical concepts but rather *everyday folk concepts*. They define emotion through its three expressions: emotional behaviour, emotional physiological change and emotional experience (subjective feelings and interpretations). Emotion, they say, is the pattern among these three events. This 'folk theory' of emotional development includes the concept of 'scripts' for each emotion.

The emotional brain is associative, laying down memories of events in terms of the context (the hippocampus) and the emotional charge (the amygdala) (Goleman, 1996). Abelson (1981 cited in Bullock and Russell 1986, p.210), states that emotional scripts are created 'in which events unfold in order' and which contain 'prototypical causes, appraisals of the situation, physiological reactions, feelings, facial expressions, actions and consequences' – thus creating an emotional meaning. The identification of a situation as 'frightening', for instance, will be made by comparison with a person's current 'fear script'.

The earliest such scripts involve the dimensions of pleasure or aversion and arousal or non-arousal created from combining subjective experience with perceptions of the environment, particularly the words, sounds and actions of the caregiver. The developmental task is one of expansion and differentiation, creating emotional scripts of increasing subtlety and variety. For this to happen, there must be an increasing range of emotional situations to experience and learn from.

There is some slight discrepancy in infant studies about what basic emotions are first differentiated. In Developmental Drama I have tended to focus on developing awareness and understanding of: *happiness, anger, sadness* and *fear*. All of these emotions have been identified in infants under the age of three. Feelings of fear evolve initially out of the startle response also known as surprise, by the building up of associations in the emotional memory on the basis of unpleasant experiences resulting from surprises. I also include the feeling of *love*. In my research, I found no mention of this emotion in infants. Perhaps it is subsumed in happiness. Perhaps it is considered difficult to identify in infant responses. Attachment, however, can be identified, and Sylva and Lunt (2000) refer to this as love. The breaking and re-making of attachments is something our clients will have to go through many times in their lives. And it is love, at its most highly developed level, that transforms empathy into universal compassion – which has been referred to as the ultimate in emotional intelligence (Goleman 2003).

How does the developing child create emotion scripts? Bullock and Russell (1986) suggest four stages and three sources. The stages of script development are:

1. Perception of gestures, facial expression, tone of voice, posture, etc.

2. Finding meaning in these perceptions – using their mother's response/behaviour as a guide to their own response/behaviour.

3. Associating these meanings to the contexts in which they occur (the language of emotions becomes important here – beginning to label).

4. Construction of emotional scripts – associating multiple elements together – combining temporal and causal sequences – attaching labels supplied by the culture.

The sources for emotion scripts are:

- The surrounding community who label some episodes with particular emotions.

- Caregivers who interpret the child's own emotions and those of others around them.

- Stereotyped narratives the child is exposed to (stories, films, etc.).

The above shows the importance of social experience in this process. The development of emotion and emotional communication is 'a coordination between social experience and maturation' (Buck 1986, p.121).

Goleman (1996) cites a project in California that demonstrates the value of stories in teaching emotional literacy. He also emphasises that, due to the associative and symbolic nature of the emotional mind, 'similes, metaphors and images speak directly to the emotional mind as do the arts' (Goleman 1996, p.294). He includes rituals, dreams and myths as being in the language of the emotional mind. For people with profound and severe learning disabilities, drama should be an ideal medium for developing emotion scripts, so long as the experiences are accessible to them and there are people present who can reliably interpret the client's responses.

THE NEEDS OF PMLD/SLD CLIENTS IN TERMS OF EMOTIONAL DEVELOPMENT

There is a bewildering array of conditions and syndromes that can interfere with the development of emotional intelligence in our clients. The challenge in Developmental Drama is to create new circumstances appropriate to development that can actually be assimilated.

To develop their emotional intelligence, a person needs to perceive, attend to and categorise emotional expressions. They also need to have their own emotional expressions perceived, and contingently responded to. This includes the reciprocal mirroring, exaggerating and expanding of these expressions. For this to happen, the responses of others need to be made accessible to them. From attention, perception, mirroring and responding, can develop labelling – a shared language for emotion. Setting the language within a repeatable narrative can then create meaning.

Ego development – having a concept of self as separate from others – is a process assisted by the infant's observations of their effect on objects and people in their environment (Schaffer 1996). Visual impairment and physical disabilities can significantly reduce the amount, range and quality of opportunities to make those observations, delaying and distorting self-concept. A self-concept, consisting of attitudes, feelings and beliefs about oneself when extended to acknowledging others as selves – similar but different – is essential to empathy, as previously mentioned. A child's use of the word 'no' has been described as 'the essence of self-representation' (Warren 1994, p.291). It shows that the child has some locus of control, a sense they can influence events in their life. Therefore, providing PMLD/SLD clients with choice and respecting their right to refuse, whenever possible, supports their growing sense of self.

The sharing of attention between oneself, an object (or event) and another person is known as the triangle of reference (Webster and Roe 1998). Also referred to as joint attention (Nafstad and Rødbroe 1999), this interactive sharing is essential in developing communication, including emotional communication, by bringing experience and language together. Sensory impairment and difficulties in sensory processing create problems for both partners in this interaction, making cues and intentions difficult to read. Both the object, or event, and the responses of the partner, may not be sufficiently accessible to a person with PMLD, more so if they also have sensory disabilities.

Due to an emphasis on other kinds of basic needs, some carers are not sharing themselves with the multiply disabled people in their care by talking about their own thoughts and feelings. Without this, it must be very difficult for a person with profound or severe multiple disabilities to create an inner representation of another. A difficulty in perceiving the emotional states of themselves and others, combined with a lack of engaging in symbolic play, can create an 'autistic-like syndrome' in some visually impaired people (Hobson *et al.* 1997). Many people with PMLD/SLD, who also have sensory impairments, can behave as if they were autistic because of their difficulties in making sense of changes in their environment and having a real sense of the responses and experiences of others.

The emotional environment is a social environment, involving communication. Emotional development can only take place in a social context. The concept of a zone of proximal development, mentioned earlier, indicates that a multiply disabled person, with support from others, can engage in and learn from a situation that they could not learn from on their own. We know that very young children can learn about dramatic play when older siblings engage them in their own dramatic play. Ferguson and Buultjens (1995) found that older children were important in encouraging play in young blind children. This indicates that our clients could benefit from a scaffolded approach to emotional development, where they are playfully drawn into engaging with a dramatic scenario, providing it is sufficiently accessible to them. When supporting clients within Developmental Drama, we need to both relate with them like a responsive mother and play with them like an older sibling. What then happens within this relationship needs to be carefully structured for maximum accessibility and assimilation.

5

SUPPORT STAFF IN DEVELOPMENTAL DRAMA

Dramatherapists can work either with individuals or with groups. In Developmental Drama you work with both of these *at the same time*, using the dynamics of the mother/infant relationship within the group context. Dramatherapists who work with PMLD/SLD clients know very well that support staff are essential and influential members of the dramatherapy group. Creating a safe and trusting relationship with someone who is multi-sensory impaired is a long task (Aiken *et al.* 2000) which the support staff have a head start on. If they are to work effectively with the dramatherapist to promote development within drama, they need to be clear and confident about their role in the process.

Depending on the context, they will already have some kind of established role with the clients, generally a caring role, or within educational settings, a learning support or teaching assistant role. There are also especially trained staff called 'intervenors', who act as a bridge between a multi-sensory impaired person and the environment. Because both distance senses are affected in MSI, it is essential literally to intervene because otherwise the person would be unable to access the environment in any meaningful way. Generally, intervenors are good at adapting to the Developmental Drama setting because they do not see themselves primarily as 'carers'. Their main concern is enabling action, understanding and interaction. When a person sees their main role as a caring one, the potential for colluding with disability can increase.

It is essential that support staff re-envisage their role when it comes to Developmental Drama. In their interactions with the person they are supporting within sessions, not only will they be assisting play development by playing with them, they will actually be helping the client to organise their experience and their thinking about the experience through the language (words and/or signs) they use with the client (Vygotsky 1986). Support staff need to feel confident, but also be open to change – to new ways of working, new experiences and new responses from the clients. This can seem a tall order in some settings, and may take some time to develop with the support staff – but it is necessary. The dramatherapist needs to consciously take on the task of bringing staff in the session on board by understanding and empathising with them, providing them with information and support and role-modelling for them. My experience has been that, if you begin by respecting them and acknowledging their skills, if you show them that what you are trying to do is enjoyable and actually helps the people they care for, support staff will respond to the new role requirements within Developmental Drama. They need to learn to trust the dramatherapist who works in a way that is different from the normal routines of the institution. They need to be given time, clarity of information and on-going support and encouragement. Just like the clients, support staff need to feel safe enough, motivated enough and confident enough to engage in an interactive and emotionally challenging environment.

THE ROLE OF 'SUPPORT-ACTOR'

I initially started working within the Elemental Play approach described in Chapter 8. Largely through role-modelling interactive play with clients, I gently drew my staff into the play. This was inspired by the play that happens naturally within the mother/infant relationship. It has much in common with what is now called Intensive Interaction (Caldwell 2005; Nind and Hewett 2005), but was formulated separately within my own dramatherapy context.

At first the support staff seemed to view me as well meaning but eccentric. I would bring them once a week, every week, into the drama studio, provide a range of sensory props, materials and sound effects within an overall theme, get down on the floor with the clients and play. But soon the staff became aware of the increased pleasure and motivation the people they cared for were showing in the sessions. The proof of the pudding was in the eating, and staff began to play with the clients too. I never insisted they do anything they felt uncomfortable with. I always explained to them beforehand what I would be doing and why. This requires the dramatherapist to hold a balance of confidently resting in their own role and expertise while respecting and including the expertise of the support staff. I asked their advice on the setting up of sessions – who worked well with whom, how people could be made most comfortable, etc. And I always spent time at the end asking for their observations, feelings, responses and ideas regarding what had happened in the session.

Note that I include their feelings. How support staff are feeling will influence the responses of people with PMLD/SLD and should be talked about (Nind and Hewett 2005). In their book on developing communication with people with multi-sensory impairment, Nafstad and Rødbroe (1999) expressed the need for co-creative relationships. What the staff, clients and I were engaged in was a co-creative relationship – we were explorers on a journey which we created together as we went along. I was the 'leader' and had some vision of where we were going and what we were looking for, but I made it clear that I relied on their expertise and understanding of the clients. I also made it overtly clear to the support staff that the clients were co-creators with us. We were all part of the dramatherapy circle, and the clients' responses were considered valuable information that helped shape what happened next.

In 2003 I took some of my evolving approaches to dramatherapy with multiply disabled visually, impaired young adults to a specialist MSI unit to see how children with both visual and hearing impairments might respond. As this project was time-limited, I knew I had to bring the staff on board quickly, and it was then that I created my basic idea of the 'support-actor' role. Working with groups for many years, and supporting others who work with groups, has taught me that people respond well when given what they consider to be a valuable role within the overall group task. So I made the task and the role as clear as possible by sharing with them my vision through an information sheet.

THE ROLE OF SUPPORT-ACTORS IN DEVELOPMENTAL DRAMA

Support-actors are vital in enabling people with MSI (multi-sensory impairment) or MDVI (multiple disability and visual impairment) to access the medium of drama. In an educational setting, for the most part these will be learning support workers who know the learners well and can easily fulfil the role. (Volunteers and students on placement also make an excellent job of it: drama students, arts therapy students and occupational therapy students, etc.)

The role of learning support worker is not just about supporting learning and attending to physical care needs. It is also about enabling the learner to access a wider variety of roles in life. It is about enabling the person to *be* in ways other than the role of passive recipient. Some of these roles might include:

- being a group member
- being a musician
- being a friend
- being a helper.

All roles require counter-roles, someone to 'play' with. Learning support workers need to be (and usually are!) flexible in their ability to role-play. They need to play a variety of different roles with their learner, as the main way of enabling the learner to play different roles. You can't do it to them, or for them, you literally have to do it with them.

Within drama it is about enabling the person to be an actor and, through acting, access new roles for themselves. In this context the role of learning support worker becomes the role of support-actor. You are trying to support them to *be actors* – to take an active part in the drama, at whatever level they can - by *being an actor* yourselves. To do this you need to:

- be aware of the 'script' before the session

- interpret the story for your actor (learner) in as dramatic and fun a way as possible - Repeat key words and phrases. Exaggerate sounds, signs and gestures

- describe and label the emotions occurring both in your actor and in others around them - The Beast is angry! Are you feeling frightened?

- pick up on expressions (sounds or movements) that your actor makes and treat them as intentional contributions to the action whenever possible

- enter into the drama yourselves - go into a dramatic role taking your cues from the director

- maintain a sense of something special happening. The dramatic space is a kind of magic space

- enable your actor to access props, costume and role

- relax and enjoy the event!

I went through the sheet with them and made sure they understood and were happy with what it contained. I have used this sheet in different formats ever since, and it can be adapted to fit settings other than educational ones.

I also created a simple feedback sheet to enable staff in the session to provide me with written observations and feedback. These are useful for understanding more about what is going on both for the staff and for the clients they are supporting. Because the responses and communication of multiply disabled people can be very subtle and individual to the person, it is not possible for the dramatherapist to pick up on them all and also facilitate the session. Time needs to be allowed for the completion of this written feedback within the boundaries of the session time. It is integral to the session, not something tacked on at the end. The main areas of feedback are:

- How was the actor at the start of the session?

- What did the actor most positively respond to (like), and how did they communicate this?

- What did the actor most negatively respond to (dislike), and how did they communicate this?

- What other new or significant responses, contributions, were made by the actor during the session?

- How did the actor seem at the close of the session?

- How did you feel as support-actor?

If there are specific objectives a client is working on, these can be added to the sheet. Support-actors can be unsure if what they are writing is what you 'want'. We can look at how to help them with this in the section on 'Endings' in the next chapter.

Note that I am referring to the clients as 'actors' and myself as 'director'. Of course, I acknowledge the inspiration of other dramatic forms like psychodrama, forum theatre and playback theatre in using language like this. I did it intentionally to help the staff really feel they are a part of a dramatic experience, unique within their working life – one that is not simply another aspect of their caring role, but a new role that uses and extends the skills they already have. I also wanted them to see the clients in a new light – as capable of dramatic action. For the most part it has worked, with on-going, persistent encouragement from me to help them take on this different way of being.

As with my first forays into interactive play described above, the main support to this process has been the staff witnessing for themselves how the clients begin to respond in new ways within the drama. A staff member who supported an emotionally sensitive MDVI client in one of my Interactive Theatre groups (see Chapter 10 on Interactive Theatre) was convinced that her actor would not be able to tolerate the emotional stimulation and challenges that are presented in this kind of work. Later she told me how surprised she had been by his patience and high levels of attention in the sessions, as well as his willingness to interact with the characters within the drama. The things that the support staff and I have witnessed within Developmental Drama sessions are difficult to quantify but include:

- spontaneous connections between peers

- profound moments of group focus on one person, sound or event

- unexpected, appropriate vocal or verbal contributions from individuals that are just right within the moment

- people who suffer from chronic physical tension simultaneously experiencing deep physical relaxation and mental alertness

- a sense that, in one hour, we have together been transported somewhere else entirely, without ever leaving the room

- moments of laughter and excitement that are felt and shared by the whole group.

When support-actors are actively involved in the sessions, they begin to fulfil the potential of really developing play in the way that primary carers and older children do with infants. They need to involve themselves in the pretence to enable their actors to do the same. Their participation and vocal responses help to build the atmosphere and support the feelings aroused by the drama. By, for instance, convincingly saying to their actor, 'I'm frightened! I don't like that noise! We need to hide!' they will be drawing their actor into the experience. They will instinctively know to emphasise the key words, like 'frightened', 'noise' and 'hide', and then follow with the actions of covering themselves and their actor with a sheet and holding tightly onto them while the 'noise' goes on around them. A high level of involvement like this will be easier for some staff than for others. Over time it can be built up in whole groups of staff. Lots of patience, clear direction and positive role modelling from the dramatherapist are required. Once support staff begin to really use the skills required of a support-actor, they will also begin to see that these skills can be used outside of sessions too.

There are, of course, many other issues around the use of support staff in sessions, such as the dynamics between staff members, internal institutional politics, the degree of support the institution offers the dramatherapist and the quality of communication within the institution. These kinds of issues arise when working within institutional settings in general. One common issue when working with PMLD/SLD clients is about what the ratio of staff to clients should be in the session. If the clients are profoundly disabled and have sensory impairments, it is best that they are supported one-to-one, and that the dramatherapist is extra to this number. This will enable the dramatherapist to maintain an overview of the session, really observe the responses of all the clients and work at the development of new skills in the staff. Sometimes I have been able to achieve this, but not always. In my experience with PMLD/SLD, the very minimum requirement is for staff to be working with no more than two clients at a time, with the dramatherapist included in this ratio. With this level of support the group should be small, no more than six clients with three staff, including the dramatherapist. With any lower ratio than this, there will be an insufficient quality of interactive relationship happening for clients to really be able to move on developmentally.

Another important issue that often comes up is the difficulty of consistency concerning the staff in sessions and who is supporting whom. The ideal is that it is always the same staff members in every session and they work with the same client each time, but we all know this is almost impossible to achieve. Still, it is what I ask for and continually work towards within the institution where the sessions happen. Having this consistency enables the important relationships to develop and strengthen between the dramatherapist and the support-actors, and between the support-actors and their actors. It enables new skills and trust in the process to really grow. However, this kind of consistency will not always be achievable, and it is important for the dramatherapist to remember not to direct their frustration about this at the support staff themselves, but to keep negotiating about it with the institution. When new staff come in at short notice, they need to be welcomed, informed and supported as best as possible and be drawn into the fun of the session. The dramatherapist can more easily do this if they trust the containing structures in the session.

6

STRUCTURES USED IN DEVELOPMENTAL DRAMA

The essential aspects that make Developmental Drama effective are:

- Approach: holistic, process-orientated, playful and grounded in developmental theory.

- Relationship: based on trust, with familiar others, interactive and flexible – open to change.

- Structure: activities within the dramatic medium that are designed specifically to develop communication and emotional intelligence, and are scaffolded carefully according to the needs, abilities and developmental levels of the clients.

The dramatic structures used in sessions are fundamental to how Developmental Drama works. They relate to the ways in which people with multiple disabilities and sensory impairments are able to make sense of their world. We can think of these structures in terms of what I call 'The 3Rs' – ritual, repetition and rhythm. The 3Rs are actually interconnected as we will see below, but to understand their relevance for people with multiple disabilities and sensory impairment we need to look at another R – routine.

The use of 'routines' is an essential means of enabling people with multiple disabilities and sensory impairment to make sense of their world (Aiken *et al.* 2000). When their distance senses are impaired or difficult to process, routines enable people to turn their chaotic and unpredictable environment into chunks of activity where they can begin to anticipate what is going to happen next to them and around them – and what is expected of them within this. Activities such as getting dressed are structured into sequenced steps. It is a scaffolded structure. Within the activity the person is supported by others but, as they gain skills and confidence, they are encouraged to participate more and more.

People with multiple disabilities and sensory impairment respond best when the day and the week are organised through routines. Communication systems often focus on an individual's routines. This includes routine relationships as well as activity routines: this person does that activity with me – I am with this person at this time or in this place. Routines are essential as containers in which people with multiple disabilities and sensory impairment can be held, feel safe and develop. When routines are broken or incomplete, without reference to the developmental needs of the person, and particularly without sufficient warning or discussion, it can elicit a fear response which may well be expressed through anger and challenging behaviour. The disturbance of a routine could be viewed, and may be experienced, as a betrayal of trust, however unintentional or however small.

These routines are not meant to be rigid and unchanging, but to be seen as flexible scaffolding on a living and growing structure. Providing sufficient aspects of a scaffold are in place for the individual's requirements, it is possible to build in new aspects which can enable new skills to be learned and help the person develop a greater tolerance of the inevitable unpredictability of daily life.

THE FIRST R: RITUAL

Ritual is one of the early roots of drama. Essentially, ritual structures are made up of sounds, words and/or actions that are specific, can be repeated and are meant to carry a person or a group of people from one state of mind or being into another. Rituals can vary along a wide spectrum from the mundane and everyday to the religious and highly esoteric. They can be social or personal. All of us probably have personal rituals that help us in the morning to get ready to face the day or at night get ready for sleep. Ritual is about enabling change to occur. Its goal is transformation. It is more than routine (also made up of sounds, words and/or actions that are specific and can be repeated) in that it resonates with a sense of special significance that affects us emotionally and psychologically. Ritual can have a capacity to provide a powerful sense of social inclusion, and it can also help contain situations or experiences that may otherwise feel overwhelming. Rite of passage rituals have these qualities.

Ritual activities are repeated each session within Developmental Drama, both as a means of scaffolding experiences and as a means of enabling clients to move in, through and out of those experiences. The ritual structures do not have to be elaborate or even highly dramatic to be effective – but they do need to be designed to create the changes necessary. I use ritual structures throughout a session to achieve different tasks such as: establishing the dramatic space, acknowledging and welcoming all the clients, preparing clients for the emotions that are going to be focused on in the session, taking the group into the story, ending the 'action' part of the session and closing the session.

Beginnings and endings are important. They should be the same for each session. Through ritualising beginnings and endings, a very holding container is created for the rest of the session. The containing sense of the 'known' allows the clients to tolerate the 'unknown' things that can and will occur within the rest of the session.

THE SECOND R: REPETITION

Within Developmental Drama do not be afraid to repeat, repeat and repeat again. Repetition is essential in developing anticipation and enabling the group (both actors and support-actors) to participate more fully over time. You need to be aware of what you are choosing to repeat and why. Key words, signs and repeated phrases are important. These need to be continually repeated in sessions and connected with an action, person, object or sensory experience. This repetition helps the client to build a sequence for the experience, and language by which they can begin to understand that experience. It is language that enables meaning. The clients do not have to be verbal to achieve this. Remember that receptive understanding of language can far exceed expressive language in a person with PMLD/SLD.

Each session is a repetition of the previous one, with some small changes or developments. Contained within the repeated known will be some new surprise, some new challenge. Think of how small children like to have the same game or the same story repeated over and over and over again. In Developmental

Drama this pleasure in repetition is paradoxically used to enable the clients to be receptive to change. The repetition inherent in ritual can provide the same benefits as routines for people with multiple disabilities and sensory impairment. However, compared to routines, ritual processes give a sense of heightened significance to what it taking place and hold the potential for transformation.

Even within repeated rituals, you need to build in the potential for spontaneity.

As stated above, rituals are actually about change, not about staying the same. The spontaneity in a ritual warm-up lies in the personal processes happening, for instance in the way you play with what the clients present through their responses. The basic environment, sounds and actions are repeated, but the whole quality of a warm-up can vary from one session to another, depending on the in-the-moment interactions with actors and support-actors.

THE THIRD R: RHYTHM

The repetition of something rhythmic is enjoyable and can enhance the ritual effect of some activities. One of the best ways to work with repetition dramatically is through rhythm. Rhythm supports the language used in sessions, both verbal and sign language. I have worked with several 'non-verbal' people who were able to sing songs and/or hum tunes, but could not speak. The rhythm needs to be kept simple. It can be percussive (clapping, drumming, etc.), it can be through verbal chanting or a combination of both. When using chants, equal emphasis is placed on each syllable and an equal space is provided between syllables with a pause between phrases or sentences. The pace of rhythm or a chant should be exaggeratedly slow, to enable the maximum possibility for clients to join in.

Rhythm has the ability to provide momentum and carry a group to a place of climax, enabling the clients to experience the building up of tension and excitement to a threshold point where it is released – a simple catharsis. They learn to move from one emotional state to another and back again with ease. Even when their hearing is severely impaired, rhythmical movement and, if possible, percussive vibration will help to hold a person's attention and connect them to the activity happening. Hearing impaired clients can be placed on resonance boards to allow them greater access to rhythm in sessions (Brown 2003). Be careful about beating on a drum or a resonance board too close to someone who is wearing hearing aids.

CREATING THE SPACE

The space that the clients enter into, where they will become actors, needs to be a prepared space that immediately indicates something about what is going to happen. They enter an event. It should look, sound and feel the same at the start of each session – the space itself is a cue to indicate what is happening or about to happen. There might be a sound (waves on the shore) or there might be a smell (the scent of roses created by spraying rose water). There might be a bright object like a rainbow parachute in the centre of the room. Think carefully and creatively about how you want to set the scene. Make it simple and accessible. The chosen sensory cue should be relevant to a main focus within the sessions. Perhaps it relates to the theme or story the group is working with or to the warm-up they always do to start. All other sensory distractions are minimised.

The ideal is a dedicated drama space, with the potential for blackout and spotlighting. I use spotlights to light up the area within the circle of actors and support-actors and then sit or stand in the middle of this circle of light. The dramatherapist needs to remember that their voice and their presence are important cues to the clients that they are in the drama space. Many people with visual impairment have some available sight. If they have any functional vision, they will see what is lit up within their visual field inside the circle of light. The action happens in the light. Anything outside that will disappear for them, minimising distractions. Clients need to be positioned so that no one's available vision is hampered by glare (from lights, reflective surfaces or windows) or too much shadow.

If you are not able to work in a dedicated drama space, do not despair. Clear your space as much as you can. You can use sheets to cover cluttered corners and surfaces – plain dark sheets are better than white or patterned sheets. The aim is to reduce anything that will distract the senses from what you want them focused on, and to support the maximum use of what functional senses the clients have available to them.

Protecting the space from intrusion by others and also by external sounds needs to be considered as well. Communicating the need for this to the institution and to others within it can be an on-going task for the dramatherapist. It may never be perfect but, by persistently engaging in dialogue about the work you are trying to do, headway can be made. You also need to be creative in your own thinking about this. When I ran a group for adults with PMLD at a day centre for adults with learning disabilities I was asked not to close the door. This seemed non-negotiable and, unfortunately, it enabled ambulant services users who were not part of the group, as well as staff, to come into the space and disrupt the atmosphere of the group. A simple red ribbon hung across the doorway during session time successfully prevented this happening!

It is valuable for each client to begin in the same place in the space every time. This is another cue to help them orientate themselves. Beyond what is essential for the start of the session, I do not engage in any unnecessary, extraneous conversation with staff as clients arrive, and I discourage them from chatting with each other as well. I leave a 'script' for the session at each support-actor's place, with anything they especially need to be aware of highlighted. If a discussion with the staff as a whole is called for, and there has not been time before the session, I wait until everyone has arrived. The discussion then happens before the first warm-up. The focus in this pre-session time needs to be on preparing the actors to be present and ready to begin the session.

A drum can be used to create an atmosphere of expectancy by beating out a slow heart-beat rhythm as the clients enter. They can hear this before they even come into the room – it is a cue for them that they are about to enter the dramatic space. As it is unlikely that the clients will all enter the room at the same time, I sometimes allow people who have arrived early to individually have a little go at exploring the drum by feeling it resonate as I beat it, or by having a go beating it themselves. But it is important to maintain the sound of the heart-beat as much as possible to cue in those who are still arriving.

WARMING UP

Warm-up activities are always a good investment. Take your time with them. The more you prepare the clients, the better use they will be able to make of the rest of the session. With PMLD/SLD clients, there is nothing wrong with spending most of the session on warm-up activities, especially when you first begin working with a group. When warming any client or group up, the dramatherapist needs to consider what they want to warm them up to. I can use as many as three or four different warm-ups in a session. In Developmental Drama the first thing is to warm the client up to simply being in the space itself. Partly that is achieved by preparing the space and creating the initial atmosphere as discussed above. Once everyone has arrived, the individuals need to be drawn into the collective group. The drumming warm-up described below is designed to do just that. There are many other possible warm-ups that can be adapted to the needs of people with multiple disabilities and sensory impairment including parachute games, songs with the potential to use each person's name, name games, etc. If it is simple, enjoyed by the group, age-appropriate in the use of language and contains the 3Rs, it is going to do the job.

DRUMMING WARM-UP

When working at the MSI Unit, I was offered a warm-up activity by a teacher there that I have adapted and used to great effect ever since. It has a ritual structure that allows each client in the group to be the focus of attention, to be named and to be welcomed to the session through the use of a drum. I use a big 'gathering' drum because of its deep resonance, but other kinds of drums are fine too – the more it resonates, the better. I have a second small hand drum for the clients' use in the ritual. I begin by chanting, slowly and repeatedly in a rhythmical way, 'Who's here today?' If members of the group are signers, you can rhythmically sign the question as well. Support-actors repeat and, if appropriate, sign this question to their actors, encouraging them to call out, make a sound or a gesture in response. It is important to allow time for responses and to be alert to any effort that a person might be making to gain attention. At the initial stages of communication development, spontaneous sounds and gestures need to be interpreted as if they were intentional (O'Kane and Goldbart 1998).

As I pick up on one of the actor's responses, my chant becomes, '(Actor's name) is here today!', repeated two or three times. The hand drum is given to that actor, who is supported by their support-actor to drum the rhythm of their own name as I drum it on the big drum. I use the person's whole name, first and last, as this provides more syllables to chant. The chanting and drumming starts slowly, while the actor gets as much control over their drum as possible, and then gradually increases in tempo until the name is being chanted so fast it becomes impossible.

At that point I drum a last single beat and everything stops. I then say clearly, with no accompanying drum, 'Welcome (actor's name)! Welcome to drama!' The whole process then begins again until another member of the group responds and it becomes their turn. Everyone in the group participates by tapping, clapping or feeling their support-actor clapping the rhythm of each person's name in time with the big drum. It is important not to rush this process. Depending on the group's size, it can take up to 20 minutes at first. Once the group become familiar with the ritual and their role in it, the time it takes decreases, but don't pre-empt that.

This simple ritual activity contains many important therapeutic processes that are well worth spending time on. It forms part of the transition from not being in drama to being in drama. It affirms each group member's identity and presence, promoting both self-awareness and the awareness of others in the group. It increases attention, motivation and anticipation.

It focuses on turn-taking and helps clients become more aware of their peers in the group. It supports both pre-intentional and intentional communication. The drum itself becomes a powerful transitional object (Winnicott 2005) and provides the opportunity for the joint attention mentioned in Chapter 4. It provides an intense and enjoyable experience of heightening excitement. The more I think about this simple dramatic activity the more rich it reveals itself to be. Because it has a theatrical quality, I am more likely to use this drumming warm-up when I am working with a story than when working within the more informal, exploratory Elemental Play approach, where a song or parachute game is more appropriate.

USING A BALL TO WARM-UP

A very similar structure can be built around the simple game of catching and throwing a ball. I use a large, lightweight, colourful beach ball. It bounces well and is very visual, fun and easy to hold with arms as well as hands. Most groups respond well to this kind of ball. A small to medium-sized exercise or physio ball is also an option provided it is not blown up so hard it becomes impossible for clients to get a grip of. I begin with bouncing the ball in the middle of the circle and chanting '*Who wants* the *ball? Who wants* the *ball? Who wants* the *ball?*' The italic words each correspond to a single bounce of the ball, so the chant becomes very defined and deliberate. Support-actors will be encouraging their actors to respond and the dramatherapist needs to pick up on their responses whatever they are. A response will change the chant to, '(Actor's name) wants the ball! (Actor's name) wants the ball! (Actor's name) wants the ball!' I then stop bouncing the ball and ask the group, 'Shall we give it to her/him?' The group enthusiastically shout, 'Yes!' and I pass the ball to this person in whatever way best enables them to grab and hold onto it. The person with the ball is then encouraged to first explore what it is like to have the ball and then to pass it back to me with lots of vocal admiration from the group. I respond, 'Thank you (actor's name), thank you for the ball!' The whole sequence then begins again.

'WHO IS THIS?' WARM-UP

This game is more suitable for SLD groups who have some language, i.e. they can name themselves and others. It works well with both visually impaired clients, encouraging them to recognise the voices and vocalise the names of their peers, and with hearing impaired clients, encouraging them to recognise the faces and use the signed names of their peers. Generally the initial letter of the first name or first and last names are signed. More clues need to be provided for MSI clients, such as touch, finger spelling, etc. It is likely that you just need to support, as best as possible, whichever of their distance senses is most unimpaired, possibly backed up by touch clues. If an intervenor is with the MSI client they can make suggestions for best enabling that person to access the game.

Begin by bringing one member of the group into the centre of the circle, encouraging them to be as quiet as possible. Once they are there, begin to chant: 'Who is this? Can anybody tell?' Then encourage the person in the middle to provide a clue by vocalising, saying or signing something simple, such as, 'Hello everybody!' You may need to have them provide clues several times, in different ways with different members of the group, taking the person to them if necessary. Each actor in the group needs to name the person in the middle in one way or another. Then you continue the chant, 'This is (actor's name) and we like him very well!' Reminding the group to start with a soft whisper, everyone then chants that person's name over and over, starting very quietly and gradually building up to a shout. That person goes back and another person is brought into the middle to start the game again, until every client has had a turn in the middle. Chanting the name, building it up from a whisper to a shout, has a similar effect as increasing the tempo when drumming a name. It can be quite a challenge for some SLD clients to actually whisper while others find it hard to shout. This game will encourage the development of vocal range from soft to loud, and with it an experience of the feeling quality of the different ranges, and an increase in the expressive potential of their voices. Signers can build the names from very small to exaggeratedly large movements.

WARMING UP THE EMOTIONS

It can be useful to spend time on a ritual warm-up that introduces and reinforces the emotional language used in the sessions. This is especially important when sessions are built around a story that specifically focuses on developing emotion scripts, as in the Interactive Theatre approach in Chapter 10. I have done this through simple call and response chants, also involving signing, sound and gesture, that cover the main early emotion scripts: happy, sad, excited, angry, frightened and love (attachment). You chant each line (except the last) and the group mirror it back to you. For the most part it will be the support-actors who engage in the responses while they involve their actors as much as possible. The italic words indicate that the action is done at the same time. The words that are capitalised indicate that this word should be signed as well as spoken.

- I *clap my hands* when I'm HAPPY– and smile – mmmm! (Use your forefinger to outline your smile while making the sound.)

- I *stamp my feet* when I'm ANGRY – and shout – No way! (Use the hands as if you are pushing something away from you when shouting the last two words.)

- I *stop and stare* when I'm FRIGHTENED – and *shake!* – Oh, dear! (Use a high pitched quavering voice for the last two words.)

- I *hang my head* when I'm SAD – and cry! (Make sobbing sounds.)

- And sometimes, with people I really LOVE, I give them a gentle touch – or even a kiss! (Blow kisses.) This last line is not mirrored back by the group. Instead each support-actor uses the word 'love' with their actor, giving them a gentle stroke, cuddle and/or blowing them kisses.

Going over the emotions and their expressions each session, copying you in this way, can actually help the support-actors become more expressive with the clients both within the sessions and without, enabling a transfer of learning. This will, in turn, help their actors, by providing language to match the emotions as they arise spontaneously within the main part of the session, whether this is the actor's own emotional experience or the emotional expressions of others.

Below is another chant that explores the expression of emotion. It takes more time, but helps the whole group develop awareness of how different people express the different emotions. This chant can be used with PMLD clients, but is also good for SLD groups. Each time before beginning, review the words and signs for HAPPY, SAD, EXCITED, ANGRY, FRIGHTENED, and LOVING. The first two lines are chanted by the whole group. The chant can be repeated for each member of the group or for a different few each session.

- Sometimes we're HAPPY.

- Sometimes we're SAD.

- What does (actor's name) do when she/he's feeling (emotion word accompanied by sign)?

- (Allow time for the support-actor and the actor to communicate how the actor might express this particular emotion.)

- When (actor's name) is (emotion) she/he (mirror the actor's expression)!

Different emotions can be explored in different sessions depending on what might be happening in the main part of the session. It is vital that the language you use to label emotions relates to the communication system used in the client's daily life, so you need to investigate what system is being used. Despite the huge importance of affect in early language development, I have found over and over again that people with PMLD/SLD are not necessarily being given the language to understand their feelings. The Developmental Drama sessions may be the first time that emotions are consistently being both expressed and labelled for them. They will need a lot of practice!

Once you have warmed-up the group in terms of emotional expression, you can then go round and ask each actor how they are feeling today. Remember to *allow time for the person to respond*. The processing delay from the point a question is asked to the point the person is able to respond can vary from person to person, and even from day to day with the same person. You need to do your research on your clients to find out if there is a processing delay. Even when someone understands what you are asking, it may take them time to physically respond. If they are available, it is good to incorporate voice output communication aids, or VOCA switches, to enable non-verbal clients to have a voice in this. The most common of these is the BIGmack switch. A message, statement, sound or line of dialogue can be recorded on this kind of switch, which will be activated when pressure is used on the top of the switch. There are important guidelines for the use of these switches, and the advice of a speech and language therapist is helpful.

WORKING WITH STORY

The story is a core dramatic structure and also a wonderful container for the processes within Developmental Drama. Most, but not all, of my Developmental Drama sessions have been built around a story. Even those that are built around a theme instead of a story have a repeated narrative that holds together both the session and the whole series of sessions. It has been said that 'story is a vessel for carrying meaning' (Taylor 1996, p.58). A simple, repeated narrative can support the developing of sequencing in experiences, language and thought. A story can bring to the clients sensory and emotional experiences beyond the scope of their daily lives, providing alternative roles both to inhabit and to respond to.

I look for stories that present issues that are potentially relevant to the client group in a way that is age appropriate, meaningful on an internal emotional level and also simple enough for the clients to engage with cognitively. I usually draw on myth, legend and folk or fairy tales. These are stories that have evolved as humankind itself has evolved, struggling to make sense of the mysteries and challenges life presents. They tend to focus in on the big issues of life, death, growing up, loss, change, conflict and love. They belong to everyone and have a universal appeal. I have also adapted the stories of classic writers like Dickens and Shakespeare.

Once you have identified a story you want to use, find a single theme or issue within it to focus on and then simplify the story down to its very essence. For instance, the theme when I worked with a simplified version of *Oliver Twist* was 'being all alone versus being with others' and how people in the group dealt with this. Being completely separate and 'all alone', even for a brief time, was experienced as difficult. Being with others in Fagin's gang felt different from being with others in the Brownlow household. It also felt difficult to be pulled back and forth between them, for which we used a literal 'tug of war' experience. There is an example in the Appendix of a simplified version of *Beauty and the Beast* for use in the Interactive Theatre approach. More on how this was used is found in Chapter 10.

Working with the Anglo-Saxon legend *Beowulf*, the theme was about 'being brave' and what that might mean to the group. The development of that theme emerged as the group came to experience that 'feeling frightened' was actually an essential part of 'being brave', that courage was only really possible in the face of fear. There may be sub-themes that evolve, but it is important to always keep the main theme in mind and work around it in every session. In *Beowulf*, the group spent several sessions at the beginning building their sense of strength and 'being brave'. It was only at the end of the fifth session (out of ten) that the hint of something frightening was introduced. The next couple of sessions brought that fear to a pitch in the confrontation with Grendel and then the rest of the sessions were about remembering and consolidating the experience of facing fear and overcoming 'the monster'.

When I use a story with a group, I introduce it in each session in a similar way, a ritualised way, with three questions accompanied by the signing of key words: WHEN does this story take place? WHERE does this story take place? and WHO is in this story? The support-actors mirror the questions and their answers to their actors, or, if appropriate, support the actors to mirror them, creating a kind of call and response effect.

The WHEN question can be answered in different ways according to the kind of story, but I try to use the phases of traditional storytelling. 'Long, long ago' is useful when working with legends and 'Once upon a time' works better with fairytales and folk tales. When working with an SLD group on the Arthurian legend, *Sir Gawain and the Green Knight*, it became, 'In the bleak midwinter (shiver)... long, long ago' (right hand moving back over the shoulder twice). We then sang the first verse of this carol before beginning the action each week to help set the atmosphere. This was initially supported by simple sensory experiences of the images in the carol presented one at a time – hearing the sound of a moaning wind, tapping the hard, cold surface of an iron, feeling a lump of ice and watching the floor in the middle of the circle transformed by being covered with a white sheet. By the fourth session, the sensory images became more verbal and only the sound of the wind and the laying out of the white sheet were necessary.

The answer to the WHERE question will relate to the specific story, for example 'In Britain, the land of King Arthur' or 'In far away China'. When telling the story of *Beauty and the Beast*, I wanted to bring the story in closer to home and used, 'Not far from here!'

The WHO question again relates to the specific story. I try to keep main characters down to only three, for example 'A Man – Father, A Girl – Daughter and A Beast!' (*Beauty and the Beast*), 'A Girl – Gerda, A Boy – Kai and The Snow Queen!' (*The Snow Queen*). Other characters may or may not be introduced as the story evolves, but the ritual opening is restricted to the three main ones. The signs for each of the different characters are important cues, and they may be supported by a sound, a prop or an item of costume – but remember to keep it simple and consistent.

There are times when I vary from this basic opening structure. Because *Grandmother Spider* was a creation myth, I began it each session by turning all the lights out and declaring, 'In the beginning, all was darkness and endless space.' This was followed by, 'Somewhere, somehow, in the darkness a spark of consciousness was born!' and at that point I switched on a torch. The early sessions of the myth took place in semi-darkness, with the light gradually increasing, session by session, as the story progressed.

When using Homer's '*The Odyssey*', based around the ideas in *Odyssey Now* (Grove and Park 1996), I created another ritual structure to open sessions:

- WHERE ARE WE? At *sea*! On *a boat*! (Sign italic words.)

- WHAT BOAT? The boat of *Odysseus*! (Use a cabasa as a sound to indicate Odysseus whenever his name is spoken.)

- WHO IS ON BOARD THIS BOAT? Pass the sea drum around. Chant each actor's name in turn three times: '(Actor's name) is on the boat!'

- WHO CAN HELP US ROW THIS BOAT? Pass around the rain stick to each support-actor: 'I am (support-actor's name). I can help row!'

- WHERE ARE WE GOING? We are going on a *long journey*. We are going on a *long journey home*. We are going on a *long journey* to Ithaca – the *home* of *Odysseus* (cabasa). We are going on a *long journey* – on the ocean – across the *sea* – to Ithaca – to *home*!

We then did some 'rowing' while singing a simple sea shanty, rocking back and forth, pulling all together on a large circle of nautical elastic rope.

The big challenge for this group was dealing with the boat breaking up (a set of centrally placed physio mats) in the eighth out of ten sessions. The boat had been their safe place every session where they began and to which they returned at the end. They needed to find safety in a new place, a movement from the sea to the land – but also to 'home'. So for the last couple of sessions, while the overall structure of the opening ritual was the same, some details needed to be different to reflect this change.

A key point when using a story in Developmental Drama is to build the story up very slowly, session by session, with lots of backtracking and repetition. Always introduce the story and the characters in the same way each session. Then backtrack and repeat a good chunk of that part of the story you worked on in the last session. It's a repeated pattern of each session taking one big step back and then two steps forward. Building the story in this way promotes the development of narrative sequencing and enables an increase in active participation by the actors. With some stories we actually have reviewed the whole story as far as we know it each session before adding on the next little episode.

ENDINGS

Endings are as important as beginnings in the ritual sense because they help clients move from the special drama space back out into the 'normality' of their daily lives, from the role of actor to their usual life roles. Endings also need to support the processes of understanding what has happened in the session, acknowledging individual's contributions and validating successes in the development of new skills. There needs to be both reflection time and celebration time. This time has to be planned into the boundaries of the whole session time. Remember, beginnings and endings are important. If you need to omit something for time reasons, it should be from the middle, action part of the session, not from the opening or closing parts.

First, consider how to indicate the main action of the session has ended. Possibilities are: changing the lighting, changing the position of the group (e.g. coming into a closer circle), and/or together putting all the props and costumes into a special box or basket. However you do it, the group need to move from an active role to a reflective role, so think about what can support them to do this. The support-actors are essential in this – if they make the shift from active to reflective, the clients will too.

When working with a story I often use a cliff-hanger approach, finishing the action for the session on an emotional high. This may not necessarily be a 'happy' high – 'Beauty is crying!' 'The boat is gone!' 'The monster is coming!' When I have the potential for black-out, I switch off all the lights at the point I want the story to end for that session – followed by a moment's silence before putting on the room's ordinary lighting. For those with at least some vision, the darkness is the cue that the story has ended for the session. For those without any vision, the stillness and silence are the cues. It is important that the support-actors maintain the stillness and silence while still supporting their actor by being in physical contact with them. Even MSI clients respond to group stillness. It is possible to use another ending cue such as a single beat of a drum, but it must be a clear cue followed by stillness and silence. During this silence, preferably in the darkness, the props and costumes should be gently relinquished and removed from the circle. The first thing to be addressed at the end of this silence is how the actors are feeling now. What has just happened? How does it make them feel? The dramatherapist needs to lead the support-actors in addressing these things with their actors.

When working within the Elemental Play approach, the ending ritual often uses some of the 'with' relationship movements as described in Veronica Sherbourne's *Developmental Movement for Children* (2001), such as rocking back to back or in the cradling position with a special relaxing song that fits the theme. This re-affirms the safety of the actor/support-actor relationship after the challenges of the session, and helps to move both partners into a more relaxed and reflective space.

The ending of a session will be partly used for the completion of the written feedback by the support-actors, as described in Chapter 5. Support staff often need help to understand what kind of feedback is useful. They may know that their actor enjoyed something, but are not clear *how* they know. It is this HOW that is important in understanding the communications of the clients. You need to be asking the support-actors, 'What did the actor *do* to make you think they enjoyed or didn't like something, were frightened, were anticipating, etc?' You want them to give some snippets of observational evidence to support their reflections, such as: 'He smiled as soon as he heard the sound of...' 'She leaned towards me and snuggled in'. Support-actors can quickly get the hang of this way of recording. It has a positive effect on how they work as support-actors in the session, making them more aware of the small ways in which their actor is responding and communicating. It is also valuable information for you, as it is hard to observe the wealth of small details when you are overseeing a session.

The ending also needs to have a strong whole group element that acknowledges the participation of individuals, one at a time. Once the support-actors have had a few minutes to write, they are ready to respond for their actor, or to help their actor respond to a question like, 'What was the best thing (actor's name) did this session?' or 'What was the biggest challenge for (actor's name) in this session?' Here is an opportunity to consolidate for the support-actors the need for specific observations as mentioned in Chapter 5, by asking the 'How do you know?' question. Verbal feedback in front of the group as a whole needs to be positive and affirmative and kept to a single point if possible. The rest of the feedback will come in the written sheets. As this is drama, there is nothing like a round of applause for each actor after their feedback to the group.

The ending of a whole series of sessions needs particular consideration. A sense of completion is required, of journey's end, and the celebration that brings with it. When the group has been focusing on a story, I do use performance sometimes as part of the process of ending a group. To share with others the story you have been working intensely with over a period of time, is a kind of letting go of the story, as well as an affirmation of it. If performance is used, it should not differ much from the ritual pattern that the sessions have had all along. It is just that the group gets bigger and the story is told from beginning to end. In my experience, PMLD clients are well aware of the different atmosphere when the group opens up to a performance.

Generally this has been a positive experience, partly because the structures hold them securely enough by then to tolerate the potential distraction of this new element.

If performance is not appropriate, then a celebration session, within the theme of the sessions, can happen. This session will focus on remembering the whole story or journey from beginning to end, remembering highlights in terms of actors' achievements, thanking each other and saying goodbye.

7

USING THE SENSES

Stimulation of the senses and sensory exploration are essential underpinnings of the creative process. It is our memories of sensory experiences that are the base material for the 'images' in our imagination, while the emotional associations attached to those sensory experiences provide the emotion tone to what we imagine. When people have sensory impairments, the images in the imagination will be different than for those whose senses are unimpaired. Even when blindness is the only disability, research has revealed that dreaming becomes quite a different experience (Hurovitz *et al.* 1999). For people with MSI, the sensory information they can gather, and the images they therefore create, are likely to be markedly incomplete and distorted, and this affects their development. Think of the classic example of the blind men telling the king what an elephant is like after each explores a different part of the elephant. Each tells the king quite a different story – none of which relates to the reality of what being an elephant really is. At least these men were able reach out, touch, handle and manipulate the object involved, as well as communicate their experience and listen to the experiences of others. All of this can be a struggle at best and, at worst, impossible to someone with multiple disabilities and sensory impairment. Significant, structured intervention by others is required to enable them to maximise their sensory experiences.

People with PMLD are generally still at what is known as the sensory-motor stage of play (Jones 2007; Sylva and Lunt 2000). They require lots of sensory exploration to aid their development, but they also require their experiences to be contained, ordered and predictable, particularly when the distance senses are impaired. The structures of Developmental Drama are designed to meet both of these needs. However, working with the senses can be complex and full of issues for both profoundly and severely disabled people.

Sensory overload can easily happen and this does not only relate to people with autism. Anyone who has had difficulties accessing, processing and understanding sensory information will react if they feel out of control of what their senses are experiencing, or if they cannot make sense of it sufficiently or quickly enough. Their efforts to maintain some kind of control over their own sensory experience can take different forms, including:

- withdrawing their hands, refusing to touch something or to have their hands helped to explore or handle something

- putting their hands over their ears and/or making sounds to drown out the other sounds around them. This can vary from inner sounds, like teeth grinding, to loud crying or screaming

- turning away from what is happening, dropping, covering or closing their eyes. This can even result in the person going to sleep

- engaging in a wide range of 'self-stimulation' activities. This can be because there is insufficient sensory stimulation to hold their attention, because they need to block out what is happening and/or as a means of self-soothing under stress.

Don't provide too much sensory stimuli. Allow people to focus on one sense at a time and on one object or interaction at a time. It may not be possible for a person to be looking and listening at the same time. You need to be aware that if a person's sight is poor and they prefer to use their hearing, they may turn their head to present their best ear, drop their head or close their eyes to better concentrate on hearing. They may, in fact, be attending very well. Becoming very still, or 'stilling', can be a sign of concentrated listening.

Allow sufficient time for people to experience what is happening. Don't rush on. Give each person time to take something in and to process it. Processing time varies greatly from person to person, and can be longer than you imagine. I have known people to respond as much as a full minute after the stimulus. You won't always get this right and the support-actors can be encouraged to tell you how their actor is dealing with the pace. Given the importance of beginnings and endings mentioned in Chapter 6, combined with the need for time to experience sensory stimuli, you can see that you will need to work in little chunks – and that less is more when it comes to what you do in the middle of the session. I generally work within one hour time boundaries, and only about 10–20 minutes of that is spent on the story or active exploratory play in the middle.

Make props and items of costume minimal and focused mainly on one of the senses. You can use light reflection to catch and maintain visual interest, such as a shiny sword or a sparkly headdress. For instance, in *The Snow Queen* I glued lots of glitter to a large purple comb for 'The Enchantress' to use when combing away Gerda's memories. I recommend that you wear a plain black or white top, when working with visually impaired clients. If you are light-skinned, black enables good contrast for your hands, face and any object you are holding. If you are dark-skinned, then think about wearing a plain light top. You want the focus on your face and hands, not on the colours or patterns of your clothing. In the MSI Unit where I developed some of the ideas in this book, all staff who worked with the children wore plain, black tops. When working with volunteers in the Interactive Theatre approach discussed in Chapter 10, I ask the volunteers to all wear black for this reason. I often try to encourage the support-actors to wear a plain top for Developmental Drama, but do not make an issue of it. However, if we decide to do a performance as part of the ending of a series of sessions, I ask the support-actors to all wear black, so that the focus of the audience is on the actors and not on them. They usually respond to this!

A particular smell can be a cue to a character. In the *Grandmother Spider* myth, Grandmother Spider's 'hairy hands' (socks over my hands with faux fur sewn on the palm area) smelled of rose and geranium and Death's black cloak was scented with myrrh. Sometimes the main sensory focus will be touch, such as the feathers on a hat or a velveteen bag full of heavy 'gold'. Clients should be warned if they are expected to use their senses in a focused manner. Do not thrust a strong smell under a person's nose, make a strange sound near their ears or touch them without giving them the opportunity to anticipate and prepare themselves for the experience.

TASTE

Taste is a very important sense to people with PMLD/SLD. Eating is an absorbing and powerful experience. I have seen it used a lot in structured and themed experiences with people with PMLD/SLD, both because the clients enjoy it and because it helps their support staff feel they are 'nurturing' them and giving them pleasure. There is nothing wrong with this, except that becoming absorbed in eating can take the focus away from the main aims of the session. I do use taste experiences in Developmental Drama sessions, but generally only once in a session, and not in every session. Whatever is offered is always just a small taste – a stimulus, not a meal! You need to always check that the taste experience is going to be safe and appropriate for the individual clients.

TOUCH

Vision and hearing are known as the 'distance senses' because they allow a person to take in information at a distance from the body – to scan and understand their environment. When one or both of the distance senses is impaired and there are also other disabilities, the sense of touch becomes extremely important. It can also become a battleground, as touch intervention requires moving into a person's close personal space. One of the systems in the body that helps to transmit touch information from the skin to the brain has links with the limbic system, the part of the brain associated with the emotions (McLinden and McCall

2002). That the words 'feel' and 'touch' can be used both for sensory and emotional experiences is revealing. It is vital to encourage our clients to use their hands to explore. However, if there has been a pattern of enforced control over the hands by others, as can be the case for people with visual impairment or MSI, the emotional script for touch experiences can be negative. This is often called 'tactile defensiveness'. It can cause a person to avoid touch and/or to react in an aggressive or avoidant manner within a touch experience. This reaction can vary from mild to extreme. Some clients have an actual impairment of tactile perception or tactile processing which also leads to tactile defensive behaviour. So, while touch experiences are very important, care needs to be taken with them.

It is good to remember that we are all tactile defensive at times and towards some experiences. Touching involves risk and requires trust. When encouraging clients who are reluctant to use their hands to make movements and explore props, I recommend you initially respect any resistance. Hands are more defensive than shoulders or backs, so when beginning to move into a person's personal space and initiate physical contact, using your shoulder or back on their shoulder or back can be a good starting point. That moment when you feel a client lean into your offered shoulder can be magical, as powerful as the gift of eye contact.

Having established some relaxed trust in the relationship, objects can be introduced into the space between you and the client, or between the support-actor and the actor, without any pressure to touch, setting up the possibility for the 'joint attention' mentioned in Chapter 4. Many people with PMLD/SLD have physical disabilities that make exploring things with their hands very difficult. You need to take into account these difficulties when choosing props to use, making them easy to access, hold and handle. The props will have to be taken to them, and presented carefully, allowing the client time to become aware of the object before touch contact happens. It can be a sign of motivation or even a major achievement when a client initiates reaching out to a prop or person.

Props can continue to be presented, without them needing to be touched, until some trust and tolerance has built up. Then the client's use of their hands can begin to be supported when it is helpful to do so. It is common to see people using a hand-*over*-hand approach with people with profound and multiple disabilities when enabling them to explore and do things with their hands. The helper places their hands over the other person's hands to help them manipulate an object, do a task or make a movement or sign. When done with sensitivity to the emotional responses of the person being helped, it can work well. If there is no possibility of the person physically being able to have certain movement and touch experiences in any other way, it may be essential.

McLinden and McCall (2002) point out that the hand-over-hand approach can promote either excessive passivity or resistance, and that there is a fine line between helping and being invasive and coercive. They recommend instead a hand-*under*-hand approach to start with. Here the client's hands are placed on top of the helper's hands. The helper shapes their hands around the object and slowly makes the movements to explore or use it, accompanied with verbal commentary. The helper can slide their hands back bit by bit to expose the object to the client's touch. The time needed for this process will vary greatly from person to person. I have also used a hand-under-hand approach to do movement and signing, placing myself behind the client, with their hands and arms over mine. Support-staff may not know this hand-under-hand approach and will need you to role model it for them. As with any new skill, practice it yourself until you are confident with it before trying to teach it to others.

Even with those clients who are not particularly tactile defensive, care should be taken before making physical contact, especially if the distance senses are impaired. You need to get the person's attention first, and this is best done if you are at eye level rather than looming over them. Many people with profound and severe disabilities are in wheelchairs. Get down to their level, speak their name to get their attention, tell them your name and let them know if you are going to make physical contact, 'Can I shake your hand?' Often with PMLD clients we work lying out on mats. It is then necessary to lie down with them to ensure good interaction.

Working with PMLD/SLD clients requires you to change your level often. Learn how to take care of your back and joints. If you are going to be at wheelchair level a lot you need a suitable stool that can be moved easily. I sometimes use one on wheels, enabling me to remain comfortably at their level, and to move from person to person. Never offer to help physically lift or shift a client unless you are qualified to do so. Manual handling requires training and approval by the agency in which you are working. You may be able to access training of various kinds within the agency you are working, even as a sessional therapist. Practical training on areas like manual handling, total communication, mobility awareness and deaf awareness are invaluable to a dramatherapist working with clients who have these needs.

OBJECTS OF REFERENCE

Objects can be central to the communication system of some people with PMLD/SLD, especially where there is visual impairment or MSI. Holding the object will help the person anticipate where they are or are going, and therefore what to expect might happen. The object helps the person orientate themselves prior to an experience, for instance, handling their swimming costume, smelling it even, can help a person know they are about to go swimming. The use of cues has already been discussed in the 'Creating the space' section of Chapter 6. Not all your clients will have objects of reference. But, if a client uses objects of reference, you may want to talk with staff about what object might be appropriate to indicate dramatherapy. It is best if the object relates specifically to what the person actually touches in the session, making it meaningful in a concrete way (Park 2002). If you use the drumming warm-up, then a beater might work. In the *Grandmother Spider* sessions, because Grandmother Spider carried and shook a rattle, a similar rattle was used for a client who required an object of reference. The object needs to be right both for the person and for what it represents. It is ideal to discuss this with a speech and language therapist if one is available. Otherwise, discuss it with whoever holds the most information on that person's needs, such as the key worker, teacher or support-actor.

There are many issues around working with the senses with PMLD/SLD clients. The above information and guidelines are really to alert you to this rather than to cover every base. Remember how much these clients need sensory stimulation and exploration to progress in their development. If you go at things slowly and sensitively, you will learn by experience what helps in the particular situation you are working in.

8

ELEMENTAL PLAY

Play is fundamental to the processes of normal development, creativity and drama. They all require playful exploration in order to move the process on, whether this is playing with materials, people, situations or ideas. Simple, basic play is a good place to start if you do not know your PMLD clients well, or if they have not had much exposure to interactive play and drama. It is where I began with this client group and where I return when it is developmentally important to do so. Elemental Play, as described here, is about simple, non-pressured exploration, the kind a baby engages in with primary carers and is especially designed for clients with profound multiple disabilities. We have already seen in Chapters 3 and 4 that people with PMLD confront huge obstacles when it comes to development, including learning to play. Without structured intervention, a person with profound disabilities is not able to move beyond the world of their own bodies, especially when one or both of the distance senses is impaired.

I term it Elemental Play because it contains the basic elements of play and drama within it and because it draws on elemental themes to help provide containment, coherence and meaning. The aims of Elemental Play are to:

- develop interactive communication

- encourage personal autonomy

- engage the senses

- promote body awareness and intentional movement

- help people experience the effects of their own actions

- encounter basic natural images and themes that are universal to human experience.

Elemental Play rests in the early development of interactive communication within the mother/infant relationship. Dialogue-like patterns of behaviour between mothers and babies have been referred to as 'reciprocity'. Mothers and babies become absorbed in each other in a way that takes on the quality of a conversation with each one's contribution being influenced by the contribution of the other. Reciprocity is a basic characteristic of human interaction. Let's look at some elements of this reciprocal behaviour from the mother's side (Harris 1990; Schaffer 1996; Stern 2002; Sylva and Lunt 2000).

- *Physical contact and gazing*: Mother holds or touches the baby, bringing her face close to the baby's face, gaining and maintaining eye contact.

- *Mirroring movements*: Mother moves her head and body in response to the baby's movements.

- *Vocal mirroring*: Mother repeats and expands on her baby's vocal sounds.

- *Rich interpretation*: Mother attributes meaning to the baby's sounds, movements and gestures.

- *Contingency*: Mother sensitively tunes in to the baby's point of view, needs and expressions and responds in a way that shows she has heard and understood. This sensitivity includes knowing how much stimulation to provide and when *not* to interact with the baby.

- *Turn-taking*: Mother allows gaps in her interactions to make space for the baby's 'replies'. She creates little games that have a back and forth/give and take quality to them, or are directed at eliciting a specific response, as in tickle games.

- *Motherese*: Mother speaks slowly, using simple, repeated words and phrases, and plenty of variation in intonation.

- *Social routines*: Mother provides contextual support to enable the baby to understand her by focusing communication interactions around repeated events that the baby becomes familiar with (i.e. nappy changing, feeding, dressing, etc.) These routines provide a role for the baby within them.

- *Joint reference*: Mother directs the focus of the 'conversation' to objects that can be mutually regarded and experienced.

All of these elements of reciprocity are meant to be worked on within Elemental Play. Support-actors take on the role of 'mother' within it as described above. It is literally about one-to-one therapy happening within group therapy. It can be done simply as one-to-one therapy, but I feel that it is more effective in a well-functioning group where there is a sense of being held and a part of a bigger event, and there is the opportunity to share experiences. Reciprocity is also important in all kinds of Developmental Drama sessions, but it is the overwhelming focus of Elemental Play.

Elemental Play is best done in small groups, six clients maximum, ideally with one-to-one support, but with a minimum of one staff member to two clients. If you are not able to have one-to-one support, then support-actors will have to shift their attention from one actor to another throughout the session, which lessens the amount of interactive playtime each client has in the session. However, the potential for there to be peer-to-peer interaction can be maximised by a skilful support-actor working with two clients together.

The sessions all revolve around a simple universal theme that holds the potential for lots of simple sensory exploration. The themes I have used the most are the four elements (earth, air, fire and water) and the four seasons (spring, summer, autumn and winter). Remember the value of repetition. When working with the elements, we stay with one element for three to four weeks at a time, exploring it with more confidence each session, before moving on to another element. At the end of the whole series of sessions we go on a journey together, visiting each element in turn. When working with the seasons, we explore a different season every week, but go through the whole cycle of seasons three to four times. On the last session we visit all the seasons, one after another, focusing on the favourite seasonal experiences for each client. There are many theme possibilities. Dramatherapy students who have worked with me have come up with other themes, like focusing on different natural landscapes or on each of the four senses. The theme is a container, giving the sessions a meaningful context in which to play. It needs to create a simple, natural setting for the sessions as a whole.

What happens within this setting is largely based on the play found in the mother/infant relationship as described in Chapter 3, but has some elements of whole group work and peer interaction as well. If it is possible, have everyone come out of chairs and onto floor level in a loose circle, either sitting or lying down. This really requires thick mats or carpet on the floor. Clients may have to be carefully positioned and supported with cushions. Make certain that they are all in a position which allows them to maximise the use of their available senses and move their body as much as possible. They need to be close enough to have awareness of the others in the group, but with the scope to stretch and move as much as they are able to.

The relaxed trust and mutual awareness of mother and infant interaction is what Elemental Play is aiming for, so begin with a whole group activity that is both enlivening and relaxing. Singing and gentle movement with touch are good beginners. The use of a parachute can add a special 'lifting' experience that is universally enjoyed. Focus on and name each actor in turn. After a member of the group is named and greeted with song and movement, I like to then play '1, 2, 3, up!' with the parachute and let it float down on top of them. We all wait for them to pull the parachute off themselves or to make a movement or sound to indicate they are still there. This is reminiscent of the simple 'peep-o!' game played with infants, but can be done without going into a place where the clients are infantilised. It is a fine line, I grant you, but your tone needs to reflect your purpose, which is to provide an enjoyable, developmental, sensory experience for people you respect. I often create the space for an Elemental Play group just by laying out a colourful parachute in the middle of the mats as the main cue. As clients arrive and are helped into position, they can reach out and touch or move the parachute while waiting for the rest of the group to arrive. You can create something similar with a large piece of lightweight fabric if you do not have a parachute.

Once your opening ritual is completed you move into the thematic experience. Here it is necessary to move the focus from the group to the experience of interactive play between two people. However you choose to introduce the theme, you will begin to bring in sensory experiences which become a joint focus for each actor and support-actor together. You supply a simple narrative, 'I can hear a cold wind!' and a sensory experience (some electric fans placed around the edges of the room are switched on, or the sound of wind blowing is played on an audio machine). 'It's wintertime!' (Some pieces of white fabric or netting are placed within reach of the actors or floated over them.) More simple narrative and possibilities for simple sensory exploration are provided as the session progresses, with plenty of time in between for exploration.

What is as, or more, important than the narrative and sensory input, is the interaction that happens within the actor and support-actor relationship. At its best, the support-actor will be following any subtle lead of their actor, picking up and using their sounds and movements, while providing a verbal and sound commentary around what is happening and what the actor seems to be experiencing. 'It's white! You're touching it. I'm touching it too! Pushing it away. We're pushing it away! Yuk! You didn't like that!'

Working in this way takes skill and experience. It has a lot in common with what is called Intensive Interaction (Nind and Hewett, 2005) and a dramatherapist will benefit from an understanding of these theories and practices. On the other hand, it is wonderfully natural and easy to do, once you realise what it is you are trying to do and give yourself permission to do it. I have trained many support-actors to work in this way over time, by discussion and by role-modelling. They, too, have really just needed to understand the reasons for it, and to be given permission. It's important not to feel the pressure of 'getting it right', but rather to have the permission to play and experiment. And it should feel enjoyable and intrinsically satisfying, as all play feels.

An Elemental Play session requires the same general aspects of ending as described in Chapter 6. Using some kind of gentle, supportive movement to music or song will reaffirm the sense of relaxation and trust in the actor and support-actor relationship, and in the group as a whole. The group also need to openly reflect on and record the responses of individual clients in the session, acknowledging feelings and celebrating achievements. As it is not an overtly dramatic way of working, I generally do not use group applause to end with, but thank the group in a more quiet way.

9

DEVELOPING ROLE PLAY

Humans are social animals – we interact, and interaction implies role. Roles in the social sense enable people to have expectations of how others might behave towards them. On a very basic level it is 'turn-taking' – you do this and I do that in response, so you can do yet another thing and so on. If I am in a restaurant as a customer, I can expect to be served food by someone else. My role is to choose, order, eat and pay. Their role is to give me options, listen to my choice, provide it, clear up afterwards and receive my money. We each know our own role in our interactions and rest in the expectation that the other person know theirs. Our roles in life help us build up our sense of self. To have many roles, be flexible within those roles in response to changing situations and be able to create new roles in response to new situations are characteristics of a healthy, developing person.

People with PMLD/SLD do have roles and can engage actively in playing those roles, but they are severely limited in their role repertoire. Often that role is a recipient role, being cared for. The bottom line for everyone is survival and the meeting of basic needs. Like babies, people with profound disabilities are compelled to draw others to them in order to have their basic needs met. They need to illicit the 'carer' role in others and some people with PMLD can be quite active in how they do this. Henry, mentioned in Chapter 2, is an excellent example. His face lights up and he vocalises in a pleasant way when he hears the voice of someone he wants contact with. His big grin is very appealing and it is hard to resist going to him. Once he draws you to him, he keeps you there with his chuckle and general animated responses to your interactions with him. If your attention is drawn away he will vocalise to gain your attention again. It is clear Henry works hard to gain and maintain social interaction, playing the role of 'cheery chap' with some skill.

Developmental Drama introduces people with profound and severe disabilities to a wider range of role possibilities, moving from simple playful turn-taking towards being part of more complex interactions in dramatic scenarios. True engagement in dramatic role requires an understanding of pretence, which many people with profound disabilities have not yet achieved. What Developmental Drama does is use dramatic role to help build the foundations underpinning pretence.

ENCOUNTERING ROLE

The Encountering Role approach builds upon Elemental Play, remembering and utilising the important role of older siblings and other children in early play development. It is suitable for PMLD and SLD clients, who can experience role-play by being swept up in it. In this case the 'older siblings' are the dramatherapist and the support-actors.

A very simple story structure is used that the clients can easily begin to anticipate and feel comfortable with. Client-actors are put into role when others relate to them as if they are in role. They are given simple role tasks within the session structure and as part of the action in the drama. This approach encourages the beginnings of role-play, and introduces people with PMLD/SLD to the structure of dramatic narrative.

The aims of Encountering Role are:

- to develop awareness of self

- to experience the physical body in relationship to both the physical space and another person

- to experience having a meaningful role in a motivating social activity that includes peers

- to experience sensory images in the context of cohesive narrative

- to develop communication skills of turn-taking, joint attention, anticipation, vocalisation and other communicative responses

- to develop emotional literacy skills of attention, motivation, experiencing and expressing emotions, perceiving emotions of others and autonomy.

Remember the 3Rs as you create these kinds of sessions. Ritual beginnings, ritual ways of entering the narrative and ritual endings are all important. Be sensory, without overloading the senses. Provide simple narratives, with repeated key words and phrases. The role of the dramatherapist as narrator in these sessions is important. Your careful, consistent narration will help to contain and guide the experience for the actors and support-actors.

The narratives I have used generally revolve around a very simple journey to an imaginary setting, with sensory experiences the clients can relate to. We go somewhere. It could be a forest, a garden, a circus, a farm or a supermarket, and so on. Once there, we explore, meet someone, find something and/or do something. Then we say goodbye to the place and person and return. In some groups I have begun the journey by using a large old key to open an imaginary door. Other groups have flown on a magic carpet or ridden on a special train. All of these have their own particular sound effect, movement and/or sensory prop to indicate the transition from one dramatic space to another. In every session we travel in the same way and, although the setting may be different each time, the rhythm of the narrative is very similar. The atmosphere of a setting is evoked through sensory experiences: sounds, smells, props, costumes, etc. and action-orientated experiences: encounters, events, tasks, etc.

For example, we use the key to open the 'door' and find ourselves on a beach. After exploring for a while, a mermaid (one of the clients 'transformed' into a mermaid) arrives and takes us under the water. We find a beautiful shell. An octopus (a support-actor with some long, flexible tubing) tries to grab us! The mermaid rescues us and we return to the beach. We say goodbye to her and return back the way we came.

One opportunity to experience playing a particular role is having a client-actor take responsibility for the transitional journey: the keyholder who opens the door, the train driver who leads the 'train' or the genie who rolls out the magic carpet. This role can rotate around the group. Another opportunity is to play the person who we meet in the special place. The actor and their support-actor together act as one to create the role. In the above scenario, the support-actor needs to be as much of a 'mermaid' as their actor, and this is a great way to introduce support staff to taking part in role-play. Simple items of costume or simple props are all that is needed to indicate a role. The mermaid in this scenario was a girl in a wheelchair. She was given a lovely piece of shiny, green fabric to cover her lap and legs. A similar piece of fabric was wrapped around her support-actor. Remember, the client does not need to understand what a mermaid is. Hats can be used, but PMLD/SLD clients can often be intolerant about having things on their head. The support-actor needs to introduce the costume or prop carefully, allowing the actor to explore the costume or prop before they are expected to wear or carry it. Props and costume need to be minimal – clear and sensory, but not too distracting.

When the group have returned from wherever they have been, take time together to reflect on the experience, acknowledging any pleasant and unpleasant experiences, as well as any achievements and contributions, before going into a ritual ending of the session.

GROUP ROLE

The Group Role approach is where the group take on a role all together and go on a journey to accomplish a task. Hero legends provide perfect material for this way of working. There are also some folk or fairy tales, built around a hero or heroine, which can also be used. Group Role is a step beyond the simple exploratory scenarios in the Encountering Role approach, in that it focuses on one particular story and one particular role that evolve over time. Strong containment is provided when the role and the narrative remain constant. The whole group are in it together, facing the challenges together, growing and developing together.

The aims of Group Role include:

- developing awareness of self and others

- developing communication skills, including anticipation, turn-taking and joint attention

- developing attention and concentration

- expressing emotions and becoming aware of emotions in others

- hearing and using emotional language

- listening and responding to the story characters, particularly their emotional expressions

- developing narrative sequencing skills.

The first time I used this approach was with the myth of *Grandmother Spider* (Eliot *et al.* 1994) mentioned in Chapter 1. The group became 'The People' who travel over time through different worlds, from being all jumbled together in a dark cavern of strange noises to finally becoming real people living in our world and seeing 'Tawa' (the sun) face to face. The journey is literally an upwards one, from lying on the ground, to crawling, to sitting and then to moving in space in different ways. Each world has a bit more light than the last, and The People learn more each time about what it is to be people. Their guide on the journey is Grandmother Spider herself. As the dramatherapist, I play this role, as it is a holding, guiding role and enables me to narrate as well. This version of *Grandmother Spider* is a story about development itself. It works wonderfully well and I have adapted it for many different groups.

Other hero legends I have used are *Theseus and the Minotaur*, *The Odyssey* (adapted from Grove and Park 1996) and *Beowulf.* I have used all of these with a variety of groups, adapting them as necessary. The group are always collectively the hero, together facing the dangers and accomplishing the deeds. There are many more possible stories to choose from, but remember the 3Rs and the suggestions for story structures described in Chapter 6. Simplify the story down to those basic elements that seem to most fit your group. Build the story little by little, slowly helping the group to identify with the heroic role. Support-actors may at times need to work together to create obstacles and special dramatic effects, or you may choose to use volunteer helpers to do this. Keep reminding the group of their ultimate task or goal, so that when it comes, however challenging it might be, they will be as prepared for it as possible.

FEAR

This ultimate task may involve facing and overcoming a monster of some kind – something big, loud and frightening. Where you have a character that is potentially challenging and/ or frightening, it is important to have someone in this role who is able to hold an awareness of the effect they are having on the clients, adapt their performance accordingly and take good direction from the dramatherapist. Sometimes support-actors can do this, but I feel it is more important for them to be with their actors, supporting them to cope with the challenging or frightening experience. I usually take responsibility for this role, as in playing Grendel in *Beowulf* or the Minotaur in the *Theseus* legend, although I have also used volunteers with acting experience.

While fear is one of the basic emotions, it is very unpleasant and we try hard to protect the people we care about from experiencing it. So why deliberately frighten our clients? Fear is endemic in and existentially fundamental to human experience, yet it is the least acceptable emotion to express, partly because it is an out-of-control emotion and can be very contagious. Storytelling, drama and theatre have been used throughout the ages to contain this emotion, enabling people to experience, express and understand it. Even today horror films are extremely popular, despite the unpleasantness of their material.

People with profound or severe disabilities do become frightened. Anything that surprises them or reminds them of being hurt, experiencing loss or being in a situation that is difficult to comprehend may set off a fear response. Loud sounds, sudden physical contact, change of routine, even something mundane like getting onto a bus may trigger fear. This is especially true if the distance senses are impaired. They need to be given the opportunity to develop emotional literacy around fear as much as around any of the other emotions. Coming through a frightening situation, with some understanding of how it arose and how it needed to be dealt with builds emotional understanding and resilience. People become more able to contain the emotion when it spontaneously arises. When this happens in the company and with the support of others it can promote a strong sense of belonging.

DEVELOPING ROLE IN INDIVIDUALS

It is possible to introduce basic role play in a more in-depth way with SLD clients. One group was based around *Peter and the Wolf*, using the music by Prokofiev to support the story and the character roles. Some clients in the group were verbally able and all of them could follow a simple instruction. All clients had some degree of visual impairment. Some had a basic understanding of pretence, while others were still developing this. Each member of the group took responsibility for one of the story characters throughout the life of the group. They learned about role-play by 'being' a particular character role over many sessions, learning to do what that character did in the context of the story.

The indicators for each role were: the musical phrase for the character from Prokofiev, an item of costume, a mask for the animal characters or a hat for the human characters and a sound or verbal phrase recorded on a switch. Masks are very visual role indicators and can be frightening, confusing or even meaningless to people with a serious learning disability. Wearing one feels unpleasant and can interfere with a client's available vision. However, it is possible to use masks if it is not the clients who wear them. I use half masks that do not cover the mouth and have wide eye holes, outlined to draw attention to them. Each animal mask in *Peter and the Wolf* was worn by the support-actor, not by the actor. The actor wore the item of costume and took responsibility for the sound or phrase. Together, support-actor and actor were the role. The human characters were played by the more verbally able clients. With support from their support-actor, they were happy to wear the hats and speak the phrases themselves. The wolf was played by a volunteer applied drama student from the local university. I will go into more depth on the use of such volunteers in the next chapter. As the sessions progressed, the actors became more involved and independent in their role tasks, anticipating actions necessary within the story. It became intentional role-play on a very simple level, but to the great satisfaction of those involved. Because of the time needed to enact character roles, this did not make good performance material. However, if you have simple editing skills, it is possible to create a video or audio recording that enables the clients to re-play the experience afterwards.

10

INTERACTIVE THEATRE

The Interactive Theatre approach was designed for people with multiple disabilities and visual impairment (MDVI) to address the emotional literacy skills that underpin the development of empathy, specifically the needs to perceive emotion in others, understand the emotions and develop some language for them. As already mentioned, the early understanding of other's emotions largely relies on vision. When vision is impaired, people are at a much greater disadvantage in perceiving emotions in others and relating that expression to their own emotional experiences. Emotional sounds can be confusing for people with MDVI, and they are seldom explained or interpreted for them. The Interactive Theatre approach continues to work towards the other aims of earlier approaches, especially in terms of developing attention, motivation and communication. But it also tries to really enable emotional scenarios to be witnessed and commented on.

Within Interactive Theatre, the clients are in the role of audience member supported by another who will comment on what is happening and provide emotional support and appropriate emotional language. The audience role can allow clients the space and safety to absorb and deal with new and challenging emotional material in sessions. Working within a ritual structure, with support staff alongside them whom they trust, enables the clients to label and begin to understand the many emotions they witness and experience within the theatrical experience. This approach is most suitable for people with SLD, including those with physical and sensory disabilities, but my groups have often included PMLD clients as well. With skilled interaction from their support-actors, these clients can also benefit from this approach.

The characters from the story interact with the client members of the audience and build up a relationship with them. Whenever possible, I have tended to use volunteer undergraduate students from the local university's drama department to play the character roles. They have always been enthusiastic, committed, good at taking direction from me and very comfortable within the dramatic medium. Support staff or other volunteers can also do this adequately, with clear guidance and support from the dramatherapist. The dramatic style is one of simple exaggeration – a version of the melodramatic style of acting.

I have mainly worked with young adults (16–21 year olds) in this way, using two fairytales, *Beauty and the Beast* and *The Snow Queen*, both of which contain archetypal themes appropriate to the transition issues that face young people: leaving home, dealing with difficult feelings, changing relationships, etc. The story is simplified and focused onto the relevant themes. In *Beauty and the Beast*, there is crucial point in the middle of the process when the characters of Beauty and Beast become friends and Beast's emotional character undergoes a transformation both in voice and demeanour. From being loud and angry, he becomes gentle and sad. Beauty then brings Beast to each of the clients, one at a time, and introduces him as her friend. The combination of Beauty, with whom the clients have a positive relationship, and Beast, who they feel negatively towards, creates a state of ambivalence for clients. With support, they each find their own way of dealing with this. *The Snow Queen* provides an opportunity for clients to experience role through enacting the central characters of Gerda and Kai as well as being in the audience, giving them even closer interaction with the other story characters. Different clients can experience these roles through the weeks. I am certain the Interactive Theatre approach can be used with other age groups, providing the story and the themes are chosen as appropriate for them.

Pantomime naturally makes good Interactive Theatre. It works in the same way fairytales do. The emotional impact is lighter – less intense, but the opportunities for audience participation are increased through the traditional pantomime audience responses. I created a version of *Aladdin* especially for this client group, with story, characters and language greatly simplified. I chose to play the 'dame' role of Widow Twanky myself, because it allowed me to hold the overall process, tell the story and intervene whenever it seemed necessary and useful.

The penultimate session of Interactive Theatre is a performance of the whole story for an invited audience. The clients can then step back, becoming the back row of the audience, and allow the characters to interact with others instead of with them. This gives them some distance and a new perspective on the whole experience. It can arouse feelings of disappointment when they do not have the same intimate contact with the characters. These feelings of letting go can be further worked with in the final session, when the character actors de-role and reveal their everyday personas to the clients. They then become part of the whole group to evaluate the experience everyone has been through together. For those clients who are developing pretence this can be a time of real learning.

STRUCTURES USED IN INTERACTIVE THEATRE

This client group take time to develop skills and understanding. While it is possible to provide short or one-off experiences of Interactive Theatre, clients would not achieve any aims in terms of developmental processes. As with all the other Developmental Drama approaches, you need to remember the 3Rs and develop the story very slowly over time, using repeated key words, phrases and signs. I have included a simplified version of the story of *Beauty and the Beast* in the Appendix. Each paragraph constitutes a single session. This version of the story requires a minimum of 12 sessions to deliver, including the performance and the de-roling sessions.

Every session will require warm ups and a ritual introduction to the story. In Interactive Theatre, during the 'WHO?' section of the ritual opening of the story, the actual characters come into the circle one at a time and make their own special contact with each client member of the audience. In *Beauty and the Beast*, Father introduced himself in a very calm and precise voice, 'Hello, I'm Father,' shaking hands with them. He let them see and/or touch his feathered tri-corn hat. Beauty had a wig of golden curls and spoke to each of them in a sweet, gentle voice saying, 'My name is Beauty.' Beast wore a half mask and furry hands with little claws. He entered the circle roaring and rushing about, taking swipes with his claws at members of the audience and shouting, 'Nobody loves me!' The clients developed a comfortable relationship with Father, who would sometimes ask their advice during the story. They began to love Beauty and really looked forward to her talking to them. She would often tell them how she was feeling in the story. They felt uneasy whenever she was upset. And, needless to say, they strongly disliked the loud and angry Beast! Some of them learned to anticipate his abrupt entrance during the introduction of the story, while others had a surprise every time and required support and warning from their support-actor. The Beast character, as mentioned above, underwent a transformation, and he entered with Beauty in all of the sessions after this happened.

Because there are some strong emotions aroused in Interactive Theatre work, the ending of sessions is very important. Clients need to be helped out of the theatrical story space and into a calm, safe and potentially reflective space. All signs of the characters need to be removed and the lighting and/or arrangement of the space altered. Because the props and costume used are very minimal, this can be done quickly. Then ending rituals, as discussed in Chapter 6, can be introduced.

CASE STUDY USING INTERACTIVE THEATRE

As part of a Master's degree, I completed a case study of some MDVI clients involved in an Interactive Theatre group based on *Beauty and the Beast* (Booker 2004). I wanted to see if a series of Developmental Drama sessions using the Interactive Theatre approach would actually enable MDVI clients to access emotional scenarios in a way that could promote the development of emotional intelligence skills, particularly those skills contingent to the development of empathy as described in Chapter 4.

Three sample participants in the group were chosen as being loosely representative of the range of learners within the school's post-16 department in terms of age, gender, neurological condition, mobility, language and vision. All were largely non-verbal, had global developmental delay and visual impairment, as well as varying degrees of physical disability. The data for one of these participants had to be disallowed due to inconsistent attendance, leaving the data from two participants available for analysis.

A baseline profile of each participant was compiled using information provided by the participant's family, staff who work closely with them and school records.

The profile outlined their:

- physical/medical condition

- sensory functioning

- communication

- current level of emotional literacy (expression and understanding).

The profiles informed the design of the Interactive Theatre sessions and, together with observed responses in the first session, provided a maximum of four focus areas for data collection and analysis for each participant.

Observations of each participant's responses in eight weekly Interactive Theatre sessions were collected through the use of video and participant observation. The support-actor working with each participant recorded observed responses on a form immediately following every session. Three video cameras were set up just outside the edges of the performance space, one focused on each participant. The plan had been to video the participants' responses in three sessions: an early session, a middle session and a session near the end. But the responses to the transformation of the Beast, as mentioned above, were so interesting that I also videoed the session just after this event.

Video transcribing and analysis is time consuming, but invaluable in terms of providing the opportunity to closely observe the responses of non-verbal clients. It required approximately five hours to transcribe the responses of one participant observed in a one-hour session, and I viewed a total of 11 sessions during the research! At times, I replayed a single response several times to ascertain what might be eliciting it. To check my observations, the school's speech and language therapist also watched at least one videoed session for each participant and gave her own short written observations. The transcribed video observations and the support-actors' forms were then combed by me for evidence pertaining to the focus areas. These were each colour-coded and highlighted, enabling a 'picture' to emerge of each participant's on-going process in the focus areas.

MARK

Mark was 16 at the time of the study. He has cerebral dysgenesis of the right hemisphere with a resulting coloboma to his right eye. He has severe learning disabilities and global developmental delay. He is physically mobile and entirely non-verbal. Mark was relatively new to dramatherapy, having only experienced one series of Group Role sessions before this Interactive Theatre project.

Following the baseline assessment, Mark's focus areas in terms of his emotional literacy were:

- Attention and appropriate response to emotional cues/ language.

- Anticipation of emotional experience and evidence of association.

- Ability to cope with ambivalence.

- The occurrence of his 'grizzle' sound – a 'negative' affect vocal expression not well understood by home or school.

Mark showed a high level of interested attention during the Interactive Theatre sessions. Despite finding the demands of the hour-long sessions tiring, he willingly sat through and remained focused on all of the sessions. Normally his attention span is considered short, being physically restless and easily distracted from one stimulus to another. Even in the session where he was coming down with an ear infection, he retained a good level of attention for the important emotional events.

His support-actor had been unsure if Mark would tolerate the level of emotions he was going to encounter in the story. She thought he would try to leave if things got difficult. In fact, he never did, instead making good use of his relationship with his support-actor, looking to her for reassurance and guidance whenever he felt unsure of what was happening or how to respond. Mark responded differently to different emotional cues and expressions and his responses were within the range of being appropriate to the given emotions, showing he was perceiving them correctly. He also showed evidence of an awareness of emotional changes in the characters, developing new responses. While demonstrating he was within the 'mirroring' level of empathy development, there was no ascertaining whether he was beginning to move beyond it at this point.

Evidence for the development of positive emotional anticipation and association was shown, especially with the character Beauty. His face lit up and he made a 'happy' sound whenever he heard or saw her approaching during the character introductions at the start of sessions. Initially he developed a strong negative association with Beast, expressed through his body language, facial expression and vocalisations. This allowed for a highlighted experience of ambivalence when the two characters interacted with him at the same time in the final three sessions. Mark's ability to cope with this ambivalence progressed through these final sessions, with a growing tolerance of Beast's presence, and finally allowing brief physical contact from him. This demonstrated Mark's capacity to alter his emotional script and allow a different relationship to develop.

There was a significant decrease in the occurrence of Mark's 'grizzle' sound charted in the videoed sessions. In the final two sessions, it was basically non-existent. This decrease seemed to relate to Mark understanding more and being more actively engaged in what was happening. Observations of the 'grizzle' in the research project enabled home and school to understand this expression more fully. It seems to express his sense of being disempowered, as discussed in Chapter 7, rather than simply an 'I don't like this' sound. It can result as much from under-stimulation as from over-stimulation.

There was some additional important information arising from the video observations of Mark. Until then, the staff had not been aware of how much interested attention he gives his peers, this only coming to light on videoing him during the reflection time at the end of sessions.

The conclusions resulting from this study for Mark were that:

- He struggles with understanding and communicating his own emotions, and with understanding and responding to the emotions of others. He needs support with this.

- He has shown he will give attention to emotional language and benefits from having his own feelings acknowledged and reflected back to him through verbal labels and signs.

- He has also shown he will try to make sense of emotionally challenging situations, providing they are structured and contained enough for him.

- Drama does seem an appropriate medium for him in which he might further develop his emotional intelligence skills, when it is used in the ways that are advocated in Developmental Drama.

STEPHEN

Stephen was 19 at the time of the study. He is severely physically disabled with cerebral palsy and uses a matrix wheelchair. He has severe learning difficulties and cortical visual impairment. He demonstrates a relatively wide receptive vocabulary, but speaks only a few words, 'yes' and 'no' being among them. Stephen was comfortable with dramatherapy, having participated in several groups within the Encountering Role approach prior to this Interactive Theatre project.

Following the baseline assessment, Stephen's focus areas in terms of his emotional literacy were:

- Attention to/awareness of the emotions of others.

- Recognition and use of emotional language and expression.

- Ability to cope with delayed gratification.

Stephen displayed high levels of attention to, and awareness of, the differences between the characters, both responding to and sometimes spontaneously mirroring their individual emotional stances.

Stephen tended to deny feeling negative emotions when directly asked, but his behaviour in response to an angry Beast indicated alarm and withdrawal. He quickly took on board the transformation of the Beast character, responding positively to Beast's request for friendship. However, he expressed his ambivalence at the end by responding with a definite negative to the idea of Beauty and Beast 'getting married', instead wanting the Beast to 'die'.

Stephen consistently demonstrated his recognition of basic emotional language. He showed he was able to consider what someone who is upset might need, within the 'egocentric' level of empathy development, for example when Beauty is crying she needs a cuddle. He displayed a different attitude to positive and negative emotions. He often denied or ignored feeling angry, frightened or sad, but was very keen to join in expressions of happiness or love. This shows that repression of 'unacceptable' feelings is well entrenched.

Stephen has a difficulty with controlling his desire for the attention of others, understandable given his high level of physical disability. He can be very persistent in calling out for them, even when he needs to wait and is given the reasons for this. Stephen was always keen to have a turn within the warm-ups and he also loved interacting with Father and Beauty at the start of the story. His support-actor viewed the video of the fifth session, as well as the researcher. Both agreed that there was evidence of Stephen controlling his urge to call out in this session. As he learned to anticipate the process, Stephen appeared to become more aware of when it was not his turn. The video revealed him waiting even better in Session 7 than in Session 5.

The conclusions resulting from this study for Stephen were that:

- The appropriateness of structured Developmental Drama for practising and developing Stephen's emotional skills is apparent in his high levels of attention and motivation, even at times of obvious tiredness.

- He is expressing empathy at the 'egocentric' level.

- The data revealed his potential to develop some control over the need for immediate gratification.

- His different attitude to positive and negative emotions, while being natural, may reflect an anxiety that feeling negative emotions is threatening or not acceptable. This project provided an outlet for less acceptable emotions while allowing him choices in how he expressed them. Unable to reject the Beast to his face, he could reject him through his choice of story ending.

This Interactive Theatre case study provided evidence of MDVI clients:

- accessing the emotional states of others

- feeling calm and safe enough to be receptive to the emotions of others, even negative ones

- engaging in joint attention (actor, support-actor and dramatic action/character)

- understanding and accepting the turn-taking process within the peer group

- giving attention, and responding appropriately, to emotional language, including references to emotional experiences within the sessions

- demonstrating the processes of association and anticipation, creating and revising emotional scripts for characters and events within the sessions.

The processes of attending, perceiving, mirroring, responding to and labelling emotions were all present, making this

Interactive Theatre group experience a viable setting for promoting emotional literacy. It also provided a fuller picture of the emotional intelligence skills of the learners involved than was previously available, giving a platform for learners to demonstrate their abilities, understanding and difficulties. It is acknowledged that much of the data analysis involved interpreting subtle behaviours of non-verbal learners. Those interpretations may be wrong, and need always be open to revision. Observers do not have access to the subjective understanding of these clients. Only consistent responses in a wide variety of circumstances can confirm conclusions made about cognitive understanding. It is, however, possible to ascertain whether a response is largely positive or negative. This is, for instance, what O'Kane and Goldbart's (1998) Affective Communication Assessment (ACA) is based on. Much of the interpretation in this study was of this nature.

TRANSFERRING LEARNING

The emotional language used in Developmental Drama groups such as this is transferable to situations outside the dramatherapy session, and it is important that the language is picked up and used by others who work with the clients. In this case, the problem of transferring learning was initially addressed by a series of follow-up sessions about the story of *Beauty and the Beast*, facilitated by a teacher, two days after each session. This was further built on by using the language in on-going communication with young people, for instance in the post-16 forum, where they all gather to reflect and celebrate together at the end of each week.

The Interactive Theatre approach is not an easy option. It takes a good deal of planning and management, but the rewards for everyone involved can be impressive. Even the invited audience at the performance have been appreciative of what happens within this kind of process. If you have a local drama school or university drama department nearby, I recommend creating a mutually productive alliance with them enabling your clients to experience this kind of dramatic witnessing and the drama students to gain a very special acting experience.

11

THE STORYTELLERS CIRCLE

The Storytellers Circle is a Developmental Drama approach which has as its main aim the promotion of self-esteem, through enabling the individual client to become a positive focus of the whole group's attention. It has many layers of aims underneath this, including the development of communication skills, social skills, narrative sequencing and emotional literacy, as well as sensory stimulation. The Storytellers Circle is suitable for both PMLD and SLD clients. It takes inspiration from the practices of playback theatre, psychodrama and ritual theatre, combined with the use of sensory stories. There is a strong call and response structure throughout and all of the phrases used in the circle, except for the stories themselves, are ritualised – used every time in the same way.

The dramatherapist is both the narrator and the director of the action. Each session a different client in the group is chosen to present a story. The story will concern current or very recent real life happenings for that client. Within the life of the group every client will have an opportunity to be the protagonist and have their story told and re-enacted. The material for the stories is gathered from family members, support-actors or other staff who live or work with the client on a daily basis. They are then re-worked into a simple story by the dramatherapist to present in the session. Two different examples of such stories are given in the Appendix. The real effort that has to be made is in gathering the stories on a regular basis, so that the material is fresh and potentially still remembered by the clients involved.

I drum a heartbeat rhythm as the clients enter the space, creating both calm and a sense of anticipation. Once everyone has gathered, the group go through a ritual opening. A version of a talking stick, referred to as 'the story stick', is used ritually throughout the session to mark important beginnings and endings. A simple, smooth broomstick is fine. It is good to have one with bells attached to the top of it to add a special ringing sound when the stick is tapped on the floor. The director/dramatherapist taps the storyteller's stick on the floor three times and announces, 'Welcome to the Storytellers Circle!' followed by three more taps of the story stick. Then the director signs and asks, 'Who is in the circle today?'

The story stick is passed around the circle, allowing each individual's presence in the circle to be acknowledged. Both actors and support-actors take their turns in this, each tapping the story stick three times and saying, 'I am (name), and I have a story to tell!' Support-actors will need to give whatever support is necessary for the client to do this, possibly even speaking for them. The group answer back all together, 'Welcome (name), and welcome to your story!' Support-actors tend to quickly pick up these ritual phrases.

This is followed by a simple drummed call and response chant that brings the whole group together. I use a 'tom-tom' rhythm on the drum, one strong beat followed by three lighter beats. The director calls out a line at a time, which is repeated back to them by the group. The rhythm is repeated twice for each line of the chant and the whole chant is repeated three times. The support-actors all join in the chant, signing the key words. Actors join in some of the words or signs wherever possible.

We are the – storytellers!

We – speak!

We – listen!

We – celebrate!

At the end of the chanting, the director taps the storyteller's stick on the floor three times, and asks, 'Whose story will be told today?' One member of the group is then designated as that day's storyteller and protagonist. This choice is made by the director, in the sense that they will have had to create the story ahead of time, with material from staff. The chosen protagonist, either using a VOCA switch or speaking if possible, will announce, 'Have I got a story to tell you! Would you like to listen?'

The whole group answer back: 'Yes, (name of protagonist)! Yes! We're listening!' It is important that support-actors are speaking and signing all the phrases, while supporting their actor to do whatever they can. The protagonist then chooses a coloured ribbon from a basket full of different coloured ribbons and ties their ribbon to the story stick. Over the weeks, more and more ribbons are added to the stick, with every ribbon representing someone's story. The protagonist taps the story stick three times and the director tells the story to the group. It is told in a simple 'storyteller' way, with sensory cues to help the individual remember the event or events concerned. It is a positive, celebratory story. At the end of the storytelling, the protagonist taps the stick again three times.

Once the story is told, the group are asked, 'Do you want to hear it again?' With the group's support and enthusiasm, the story is told again and this time it is partially re-enacted, bringing in sensory props, sound effects and actions. Following the enactment, the group are invited to share any similar stories from their own lives. This is done by support-actors and may be about themselves or about another client in the group. I generally role-model this sharing until the group get the hang of it.

The group then go through a ritual closing of the circle, before a period of discussion and reflection on the achievements within the session: 'It's almost time to break the circle. Shall we thank everyone for the stories?' The ending chant is done as a call and response with signing, using the same tom-tom rhythm as the earlier chant. This time the rhythm is repeated twice in each line, but the chant is only done once.

Thank you for the – stories.

Thank you for the – fun.

We will meet here – next time.

The stories will go – on!

The session ends with three final taps of the story stick.

The very last session of a Storytellers Circle group has a slightly different structure. The beginning is the same, but instead of choosing a protagonist, the director announces, 'Have we got some stories to tell you! Would you like to listen?' The group answer as usual, and then each story from the series of sessions is told to the group. There are three taps of the storyteller's stick to indicate the beginning and three more taps at the end of each story. After each story, the person whose story it was takes their ribbon off the story stick and puts it back into the basket. There are no re-enactments this time and I have been amazed by the high levels of concentration and listening in this session, despite it being largely verbal.

To close the group the director says, 'It's almost time to break the circle. This is the end of the Storytellers Circle for now. We have told some wonderful stories haven't we? Some of us might meet again and tell some new stories! Shall we thank everyone for the stories?' The closing chant is done in the same way as for all the other sessions, but some of the words are different:

Thank you for the – stories.

Thank you for the – fun.

The story circle's – ended but,

The stories will go – on!

The whole group ends with three final taps of the story stick.

Support-actors can become very involved in a Storytellers Circle group, helping to gather material for stories, and sharing their own stories or stories about other clients in the group within the sessions. The very ritualistic structure of the Storytellers Circle supports anticipation and increases participation, and also has an amazingly cohesive effect on the group as a whole. The stories are collected into a book for the clients to keep.

12

IT'S OVER TO YOU

When I first began doing dramatherapy with multiple disabled, visually impaired young people, I felt like I was working in the dark. I was highly motivated, but did not really know how to begin, or what I was going to be able to achieve. There were plenty of doubts around in others about my achieving anything at all. The Developmental Drama approaches described in this book are the result of a long journey with my PMLD/SLD clients. It seemed that every time I started a new group, new possible ideas or approaches came into being. New challenges invite new ways of working. My hope is that the approaches described here can support the beginning of a journey for other practitioners who choose to work with clients with severe or profound multiple learning disabilities, including sensory impairment.

Developmental Drama is based on approach, relationships and structures. The approach is holistic, working with the whole person's development on many levels at once. It is process orientated, meaning that the dramatic activities are planned to support the processes involved in promoting the clients' development and improving their well-being. This requires an understanding of early developmental needs in general, as well as the particular needs resulting from multiple disabilities and sensory impairments.

The relationships in Developmental Drama are grounded in an understanding of those relationships fundamental to the early development of play and communication – those of an infant with the primary care-giver and a young child with older peers. They are based in trust, reciprocity, interaction and playfulness. The therapist/client relationship is not the only one to consider when working with people with PMLD/SLD. The relationships between the dramatherapist and the support workers are also vital. It takes time to develop mutual understanding and trust. The dramatherapist needs to respect and value the support workers, while communicating to them an understanding of new ways of working and being with the clients.

The structures in Developmental Drama are designed to enable PMLD/SLD clients to anticipate, respond and achieve. They are scaffolded structures, resting in the skills and abilities the client already has, while enabling them to realistically move beyond them in a supported, motivating social context. The 3Rs of ritual, repetition and rhythm, along with careful attention to beginnings and endings, are used to shape sessions in a way that builds confidence and promotes participation.

Some of the outcomes of Developmental Drama for people with PMLD/SLD can include:

- An increase in intentional communication and participation, both in and out of sessions.

- A greater sense of self in relation to both other people and their physical environment.

- Developments in emotional literacy, such as increased emotional language and more understanding of their own emotions and the emotions of others.

- Improved narrative sequencing.

- More awareness of, tolerance of and interaction with their peers.

- Pleasure, laughter, excitement and surprise!

So please have a go! Not everything you need is in this book. These pages are meant to give you encouragement and some starting points – guidance and structures to build on and then create your own ways of working. You will need to gain an understanding of the particulars about your own clients – their barriers to development, their needs, their likes and dislikes, how they communicate and so on. You will need to be constantly building up new resources to use in sessions like stories, sound effects, sensory fabrics, percussion instruments and sensory props. You will also need to understand the environment in which your clients live and work, its particular limitations and potentials. Within educational settings there tends to be a good emphasis on developing communication in the learners. There is often great knowledge and understanding in staff about the needs of individuals. However, there can also be a strong focus on tasks and on behaviour that is not necessarily appropriate in dramatherapy. Other settings will all have their own advantages and challenges.

Wherever you are, start small – with a small group, a simple space and a couple of willing support workers. Less is more. Elemental Play is probably a good place to begin if you have profoundly disabled clients. Development is always a slow and gradual process, even more so when confronted with the barriers of profound or severe multiple disabilities and sensory impairment. This applies to your development as a dramatherapist or drama facilitator, as well as the development of the people in your group. So take time, and enjoy being with others, playing with them and getting to know them through the play. The approaches in this book will need to be adjusted and expanded on to fit you and your workplace. Eventually you will find yourself creating entirely new approaches, which I hope you, too, will share with us all.

Appendix

BEAUTY AND THE BEAST - A STORY FOR INTERACTIVE THEATRE

THE BEGINNING

This section is repeated in every session. Sign key words, as you speak them slowly and clearly, giving a ritual significance to it all.

WHEN? Once upon a time.

WHERE? Not far away.

WHO? There lived a man, Father, who used to be rich, but now was poor.

And a girl, his daughter, whose name was Beauty.

On the other side of the forest, in a magical palace, lived the Beast!

In the Who? section, the characters come in as their name is mentioned and introduce themselves to the audience members (clients), one at a time. The next character is not introduced until the previous character has been around the whole group and left the circle.

THE STORY

Divide the story into approximately ten sessions, before bringing it together as a whole. Each section of the story is narrated and enacted at the same time. You will need to backtrack a bit on the story each session, before adding on a new part. You need to create very simple lines of dialogue for the characters to speak, with key words emphasised. These lines might simply be a repetition of the lines in the story narration. The support-actors are encouraged to sign and repeat key words and phrases for the clients they are supporting as the story unfolds. It needs to proceed slowly enough for this to happen. Action is slow and improvised, performed in an exaggerated, melodramatic style, with sound, lighting effects and props brought in as appropriate. Drama student volunteers usually really enjoy this. Characters actually speak to members of the audience at times, as well as show them props. Sometimes they might repeat the same phrase to several different people in the audience.

Father and Beauty live at home. Beauty is very HAPPY. She is happy to be with her Father. She likes her home. And Beauty loves the flowers in her garden. Father is SAD and WORRIED. He wants more money. Father decides to go on a journey to get some more money. He asks Beauty if she would like him to bring her back a present. Beauty wants a rose. Father says goodbye to Beauty.

Father walks for a long time. Soon he comes to a dark forest. There are strange sounds in the forest. Father is FRIGHTENED! It is getting cold! Finally, Father sees a light. He walks towards it and it gets brighter. Suddenly he comes out of the forest into bright sunshine! He finds himself in a magical place. He sees a big palace surrounded by beautiful gardens. Flowers of every kind are blooming! Father is very HAPPY!

Father is tired and hungry! Magical hands appear and serve him tasty things to eat! Father is tired now. He has walked a long way from his home. A bed magically appears. Father lies down on the bed and goes fast asleep. In the night there are strange noises. But Father is so tired he is sound asleep. He does not hear the sounds.

Morning comes. Father wakes up. He searches the palace for his host, but he cannot find anyone. Nobody seems to be here. Then Father goes out into the garden. He sees a beautiful rose bush. Then Father remembers what Beauty asked for. Father reaches over and picks a rose. The rose is magic! It begins to sing! *We used an artificial rose that I scented with rose oil. It played the tune 'Love Me Tender' when the stem was squeezed!*

Suddenly there is a terrible roar and a Beast appears! Father is FRIGHTENED! What a terrible Beast! The Beast is ANGRY! He says that Father is stealing his rose and must be punished! Father tells the Beast about Beauty. The Beast thinks about Beauty. He makes Father promise to bring Beauty to the palace. If Father does not, they will both be punished! Father is very SAD! He must go home and bring Beauty back to the Beast! What will happen to Beauty? Will the Beast eat her? But if he doesn't bring Beauty to the Beast, then he might come and kill them both!

Father walks all the way home again. He is very SAD. Beauty is pleased to see him. Beauty LOVES her Father. She gives Father a big hug! Beauty sees the rose in Father's hand. Father is very SAD. He tells Beauty all about his journey through the dark forest. And then Father tells Beauty about the Beast! Father tells her that the Beast is very ANGRY. The Beast has made Father promise to take Beauty back to the palace! Beauty tries to comfort Father. She tells him she will go to the palace. Maybe when the Beast sees that they have kept the promise he won't be angry anymore. Father is FRIGHTENED, but Beauty says she will go. And so, Father and Beauty set out for the Beast's palace.

They arrive at the gates of the palace. But the magic hands will not let Father come in. Father is pushed away. Father must leave Beauty and go home alone. The magic hands bring Beauty into the palace. Beauty is all alone. Her Father is gone. She is in a place she does not know, no family and no friends. Soon maybe the Beast will come. Now Beauty is very, very SAD. Her Father is gone! She has been left all on her own in the Beast's magical palace. She is also FRIGHTENED. She is frightened about the Beast! Beauty cries. Then she hears a noise. The Beast is coming!

The Beast tells her she must stay with him. Beauty is upset. She tells the Beast that Father only wanted to give the rose to her because he LOVES her. It was only one rose! She asks the Beast, why is he so ANGRY? The Beast is now SAD. He tells Beauty that no one LOVES him. He is too ugly and frightening! He asks her to stay and be his friend. Beauty feels sorry for the Beast. She sees that he is not really ANGRY and FRIGHTENING. Beauty sees that really the Beast is SAD and LONELY. She says she will stay for a while and be his friend.

Beauty and the Beast are friends. The Beast really LOVES Beauty. He asks Beauty to marry him. Beauty says she cannot. He is a Beast! The Beast is VERY SAD. Beauty is kind to him, but Beauty does not LOVE him. Beauty and the Beast become good friends. They talk together, eat meals together and play together in the lovely garden. But Beauty becomes SAD. She wants to see her Father again. The Beast lets her go home to visit. But he tells Beauty that if she does not come back to him he will die. The Beast loves Beauty very much. The Beast is very SAD to see Beauty leave the palace. He thinks he will die if she does not come back to him. Beauty promises to come back to the Beast. Beauty and the Beast say goodbye to each other. Beauty goes home to Father. Now the Beast is all alone again. Beauty is gone. The Beast is very SAD!

At home, Father is worried about Beauty. He thinks the Beast might have eaten her! Then Beauty arrives home. They are very HAPPY to see each other again. Father tells Beauty he has been ill with worry about her. Beauty stays at home to look after Father. Father is very happy to have Beauty at home again. Although she remembers her promise, Beauty feels she should stay with Father a little longer. Back at the Beast's palace, the Beast is dying.

The Beast does not think Beauty will come back. He does not think she loves him. He calls out to tell Beauty he LOVES her. Suddenly Beauty knows that the Beast needs her. She rushes back to the palace. The Beast is dying. Beauty realises she loves the Beast. Beauty kisses the Beast. There is magic in this air! Something is happening! The Beast stands up! His hairy paws are becoming smooth hands! His beast face is changing to a human face! He is not a Beast anymore! He is a man! He tells Beauty that he is really a Prince. He had been turned into a Beast by a wicked spell. The spell was broken when Beauty really LOVES him, even though he is a Beast, and she kisses him.

Beauty and the Prince are HAPPY together. They decide to get married. Even Father is HAPPY now, because he doesn't have to worry about money anymore, and he knows that his daughter, Beauty, will be HAPPY ever after.

THE END

STORYTELLERS CIRCLE STORIES

The stories are told all the way through first, before being re-told and enacted at the same time. Only one story is told per session, except in the very last session. The following are just two examples of personal stories used in The Storytellers Circle.

ROBERT'S STORY

Robert likes to make music. Robert makes lots of different kinds of sounds. Making sounds means Robert is happy! Robert would love us all to make a band! Robert can be leader of the band!

When we all make music together it will be like a big marching band! This is what a big band sounds like. (*Play Glenn Miller's 'St Louis Blues March'.*)

Robert likes drumming. Lots of loud drumming makes Robert very happy! Robert can play the drum and others can join him in playing the drum. There needs to be a lot of drums in Robert's band. (*Hand out drums and drum switch.*)

Robert also likes all the 'blowing' kinds of sounds like trumpet, didgeridoo, party blower and kazoo! (*Hand out 'blowing' type instruments and trumpet switch.*) There needs to be lot of shakers in Robert's band too. (*Hand out shakers.*)

Robert can be the leader of our band! First the band will practice and then the band can go on a march! (*Practice period.*)

Is everyone ready? Robert is in front because Robert is the leader of the band. (*With Glenn Miller in the background, the whole group will play their instruments and follow Robert around the room.*)

Robert's band is a great band! We all love music! And we love following Robert, the leader of the band!

THE END

SUSAN'S STORY

Once upon a time – in the Easter holiday – Susan went to Cornwall. She went to stay in a caravan with her friends, Joan and Ron. They stayed in a place called 'Rock'. Princes William and Harry have been to Rock on holiday too! Susan had lots of fun on holiday.

The caravan Susan stayed in was in the middle of a big field. Susan liked to *run and run* in the big field! (*Susan can get up and run around in the middle of the circle. Other actors might want to have a turn at running.*) At night, Susan slept inside the caravan. She slept on the bottom of a bunk bed. You have to be careful when you get off the bed that you don't bump your head! Susan slept inside a *sleeping bag*. (*Pass round a sleeping bag. Anyone want to try to get into it?*)

Susan walked on the beach by *the sea*. (*Sounds of waves and seagulls.*) Joan, Ron and Susan collected lots of *big pebbles*. They used the pebbles to make a big circle. Susan played on the *sand* inside the circle. (*Sensory experience with large, smooth pebbles and sand. Make circle of pebbles in middle of circle with Susan in the middle of them.*)

One day Susan, Joan and Ron went for a long walk on top of the cliffs. The sea was far below them. It was very *hot and sunny* (*signs*). Susan *walked and walked*. (*Walking in place, everyone stepping.*) She got *very tired* (*tired sounds, yawning, sleepy sign*), but she kept going.

Susan, Joan and Ron went on a boat called a ferry to the town of Padstow. In Padstow Susan walked along the harbour. There were lots of *seagulls making a noise* (*sounds of gulls*) and eating *pasty* crumbs (*handfuls of crumbs*). Susan had an *ice cream* (*taste*).

Susan was very *happy* (*taste experience*) in Cornwall on holiday in the caravan.

THE END

REFERENCES AND FURTHER READING

Aiken, S., Buultjens, M., Clark, C., Eyre, J.T. and Pease, L. (2000) *Teaching Children Who are Deafblind: Contact, Communication and Learning.* London: David Fulton Publishers.

Barnet, M.A. (1987) 'Empathy and Related Responses in Children'. In N. Eisenberg and J. Strayer (eds) *Empathy and its Development.* Cambridge: Cambridge University Press

Bombèr, L.M. (2007) *Inside I'm Hurting: Practical Strategies for Supporting Children with Attachment Difficulties in Schools.* London: Worth Publishing.

Booker, M. (2004) *Seeing With the Heart: An Evaluation of the Use of Drama to Develop Emotional Literacy in Post-16 Learners With Multiple Disabilities and Visual Impairment.* Unpublished MEd (Multi-sensory Impairment) dissertation: University of Birmingham.

Brown, D. (2003) *Resonance Boards.* Deafblind Resources. Available at www.deafblindresources.org/article/resonanceboards.html. Accessed on 9 January 2011.

Buck, R. (1986) *The Communication of Emotion.* New York and London: Guilford Press.

Bullock, M. and Russell, J.A. (1986) 'Concepts of Emotion in Developmental Psychology.' In C. Izard and P. Read (eds). *Measuring Emotions in Infants and Children, Vol II.* Cambridge: Cambridge University Press.

Caldwell, P. (2005) *Finding You Finding Me: Using Intensive Interaction to Get in Touch with People Whose Severe Learning Disabilities are Combined with Autistic Spectrum Disorder.* London: Jessica Kingsley Publishers.

133

Eliot A., Campbell J. and Eliade M. (1994) *The Universal Myths, Heroes, Gods, Tricksters and Others.* New York and London: Meridian Books (Penguin).

Ferguson, R. and Buultjens, M. (1995) 'The play behaviour of young blind children and its relationship to developmental stages.' *British Journal of Visual Impairment 13*, 3, 100–107.

Garvey, C. (1990) *Play* (2nd edn.) London: Fontana Books.

Goleman, D. (1996) *Emotional Intelligence: Why it Can Matter More than IQ.* London: Bloomsbury Publishing.

Goleman, D. (2003) *Destructive Emotions and How We Can Overcome Them: A Dialogue with the Dalai Lama.* London: Bloomsbury Publishing.

Greenspan, P. (2001) *Emotions, Rationality, and Mind/Body.* Available at www.philosophy.umd.edu/Faculty/PGreenspan/Res/er4.html. Accessed on 9 January 2011.

Grove, N. and Park, K. (1996) *Odyssey Now.* London: Jessica Kingsley Publishers.

Harris, J. (1990) *Early Language Development, Implications for Clinical and Educational Practice.* London and New York: Routledge.

Harris, P.L. (1989) *Children and Emotion: The Development of Psychological Understanding.* Oxford: Basil Blackwell.

Harris, P.L. (2000) *The Work of the Imagination.* Oxford: Basil Blackwell.

Hobson, R.P., Brown, R., Minter, M.E. and Lee, A. (1997) 'Autism Revisited: The Case of Congenital Blindness.' In V. Lewis and G.M. Collis (eds). *Blindness and Psychological Development in Young Children.* Leicester: BPS Books (The British Psychological Society).

Hoffman, M.L. (1987) 'The Contribution of Empathy to Justice and Moral Judgement'. In N. Eisenberg and J. Strayer (eds) *Empathy and its Development.* Cambridge: Cambridge University Press.

Hurovitz, C., Dunn, S., Domhoff, G.W. and Fiss, H. (1999) 'The dreams of blind men and women: A replication and extension of previous findings.' *Dreaming 9*, 183–193.

Jones, P. (2007) *Drama as Therapy, Theory, Practice and Research*. London and New York: Routledge.

Landy, R. (1993) *Persona and Performance, The Meaning of Role in Drama, Therapy, and Everyday Life*. London and Bristol, Pennsylvania: Jessica Kingsley Publishers.

Mayer, J.D. and Salovey, P. (1997) 'What is Emotional Intelligence?' In P. Salovey and D.J. Sluyter (eds). *Emotional Development and Emotional Intelligence*. New York: Basic Books.

McLinden, M. and McCall, S. (2002) *Learning Through Touch: Supporting Children with Visual Impairment and Additional Difficulties*. London: David Fulton Publishers.

Nind, M. and Hewett, D. (2005) *Access to Communication: Developing the Basics of Communication with People with Severe Learning Difficulties Through Intensive Interaction* (2nd edn.) London: David Fulton Publishers.

Nafstad, A. and Rødbroe, I. (1999) *Co-creating Communication: Perspectives on Diagnostic Education for Individuals Who are Congenitally Deafblind and Individuals Whose Impairments May Have Similar Effects*. Dronninglund, Denmark: Forlaget Nord-Press.

O'Kane, J.L. and Goldbart, J. (1998) *Communication Before Speech: Development and Assessment*. London: David Fulton Publishers.

Orr, R. (2003) *My Right to Play: A Child with Complex Needs*. New York and Maidenhead: Open University Press.

Park, K. (2002) *Objects of Reference in Practice and Theory*. London: Sense (The National Deafblind and Rubella Association).

Piaget, J. (1967) *The Psychology of Intelligence*. London: Routledge and Kegan Paul.

Schaffer, H.R. (1996) *Social Development*. Oxford: Blackwell Publishing.

Sherbourne, V. (2001) *Developmental Movement for Children: Mainstream, Special Needs and Pre-school* (2nd revised edn.) London: Worth Publishing.

Sherratt, D. and Peter, M. (2002) *Developing Play and Drama in Children with Autistic Spectrum Disorders*. London: David Fulton Publishers.

Stern, D. (2002) *The First Relationship: Infant and Mother.* Cambridge, MA and London: Harvard University Press.

Sylva, K. and Lunt, J. (2000) *Child Development: A First Course.* Oxford: Blackwell Publishing.

Taylor, D. (1996) *The Healing Power of Stories: Creating Yourself Through the Stories of Your Life.* Dublin: Gill and Macmillan.

Vygotsky, L.S. (1978) *Mind in Society: The Development of Higher Psychological Processes.* Cambridge, MA and London: Harvard University Press.

Vygotsky, L.S. (1986) *Thought and Language.* A. Kozulin (ed.) Cambridge, MA: MIT Press.

Ware, J. (2003) *Creating a Responsive Environment for People with Profound and Multiple Learning Difficulties* (2nd edn.) London: David Fulton Publishers.

Warren, D.H. (1994) *Blindness and Children: An Individual Differences Approach.* Cambridge: Cambridge University Press.

Webster, A. and Roe, J. (1998) *Children With Visual Impairments: Social Interaction, Language and Learning.* London and New York: Routledge.

Winnicott, D.W. (2005) *Playing and Reality* (2nd edn.) London and New York: Routledge.

Wood, D. (1998) *How Children Think and Learn* (2nd edn.) Oxford: Blackwell Publishing.

SUBJECT INDEX

AUTHOR INDEX